THE ULTIMATE GALVESTON DIET COOKBOOK FOR BEGINNERS

2000 Days Of Recipes: Essential Guide To Flavorful And Delicious Dishes To Transform Your Health And Well-Being, With A 31-Day Meal Plan

Grayson Emerson

Table of Contents

CHAPTER ONE

Introduction to the Galveston Diet for Beginners

The Galveston Diet has gained popularity in recent years as a potential solution for weight loss and overall health improvement. it specifically targets women over 40 who struggle with hormonal imbalances and weight management issues. This dietary approach is tailored to address the unique challenges that women face during perimenopause and menopause, focusing on hormone optimization and inflammation reduction.

What is the Galveston Diet?

The Galveston Diet is a science-based eating plan designed to support women's health, particularly during perimenopause and menopause. It emphasizes whole foods, balanced macronutrients, and strategic meal timing to regulate blood sugar levels, reduce inflammation, and promote fat loss. Unlike many fad diets that rely on severe calorie restriction or elimination of entire food groups, the Galveston Diet encourages a sustainable approach to eating that can be maintained long-term.

At the core of the Galveston Diet is the concept of hormonal balance. As women age, hormonal fluctuations, particularly estrogen and progesterone levels, can lead to weight gain, insulin resistance, and other metabolic issues. By incorporating nutrient-dense foods and avoiding processed carbohydrates and sugars, the diet aims to stabilize blood sugar levels and support hormonal health.

The Galveston Diet is not a one-size-fits-all approach. It takes into account individual differences in metabolism, lifestyle, and health goals. While there are general guidelines to follow, such as focusing on whole foods and limiting processed foods, the diet can be personalized based on factors like activity level, medical history, and food preferences.

Key principles of the Galveston Diet include:

1. **Balanced Macronutrients**: Meals are composed of a balance of protein, healthy fats, and complex carbohydrates to provide sustained energy and promote satiety.

2. **Emphasis on Whole Foods**: The diet encourages the consumption of nutrient-dense, whole foods such as vegetables, fruits, lean proteins, nuts, seeds, and healthy fats.

3. **Intermittent Fasting**: Intermittent fasting is incorporated as a tool to enhance fat burning and improve metabolic flexibility. This typically involves cycling between periods of eating and fasting, such as a 16:8 fasting protocol where one fasts for 16 hours and eats within an 8-hour window.

4. **Blood Sugar Regulation**: By minimizing intake of refined carbohydrates and sugars, the Galveston Diet aims to stabilize blood sugar levels and reduce insulin resistance.

5. **Inflammation Reduction**: Certain foods, such as processed foods, refined sugars, and vegetable oils, are known to promote inflammation in the body. The diet focuses on anti-inflammatory foods like fatty fish, leafy greens, and berries to mitigate inflammation.

Overall, the Galveston Diet promotes a holistic approach to health that goes beyond just weight loss. By addressing hormonal balance, blood sugar regulation, and inflammation, it aims to improve overall well-being and reduce the risk of chronic diseases associated with aging.

Benefits of the Galveston Diet for Beginners

The Galveston Diet offers a range of potential benefits for beginners and experienced practitioners alike. Here are some of the key advantages:

1. **Weight Loss**: One of the primary goals of the Galveston Diet is weight loss, particularly targeting stubborn belly fat that tends to accumulate during perimenopause and menopause. By promoting fat burning and reducing insulin resistance, many women experience significant weight loss and improved body composition.

2. **Hormonal Balance**: Hormonal fluctuations during perimenopause and menopause can lead to a range of symptoms, including hot flashes, mood swings, and weight gain. The Galveston Diet aims to support hormonal balance by optimizing nutrient intake and regulating blood sugar levels, which may alleviate these symptoms.

3. **Improved Energy Levels**: Stable blood sugar levels and balanced macronutrient intake can lead to sustained energy throughout the day. Many women report feeling more energized and alert after adopting the Galveston Diet.

4. **Reduced Inflammation**: Chronic inflammation is linked to numerous health problems, including heart disease, diabetes, and autoimmune conditions. By emphasizing anti-inflammatory foods and avoiding pro-inflammatory foods, the Galveston Diet may help reduce inflammation and lower the risk of related diseases.

5. **Better Metabolic Health**: The Galveston Diet can improve metabolic health by enhancing insulin sensitivity and promoting fat burning. This may lead to a lower risk of type 2 diabetes and other metabolic disorders.

6. **Enhanced Mental Clarity**: Some practitioners of the Galveston Diet report improved mental clarity and focus, which may be attributed to stable blood sugar levels and reduced inflammation in the brain.

7. **Long-Term Sustainability**: Unlike many fad diets that are difficult to maintain long-term, the Galveston Diet offers a flexible and sustainable approach to eating. By focusing on whole foods and balanced nutrition, it can be adapted to fit individual preferences and lifestyles.

8. **Support for Overall Well-being**: In addition to physical benefits, many women find that the Galveston Diet improves their overall sense of well-being, including mood, sleep quality, and stress management.

While individual results may vary, the Galveston Diet provides a comprehensive approach to health and wellness that addresses the unique needs of women over 40.

Getting Started: Beginner's Guide to the Galveston Diet

Starting any new diet can be daunting, but with the right guidance, beginners can ease into the Galveston Diet and begin experiencing its benefits. Here's a step-by-step guide to getting started:

1. **Educate Yourself**: Before diving into the Galveston Diet, take some time to educate yourself about its principles and guidelines. Familiarize yourself with the types of foods to include and avoid, as well as the recommended meal timing and portion sizes.

2. **Assess Your Current Diet**: Take stock of your current eating habits and identify areas for improvement. Are you consuming too many processed foods and sugars? Are you getting enough protein and healthy fats? Understanding your starting point will help you make necessary adjustments.

3. **Set Realistic Goals**: Determine what you hope to achieve with the Galveston Diet, whether it's weight loss, improved energy, or better hormonal balance. Set realistic, achievable goals that you can work towards over time.

4. **Clean Out Your Pantry**: To set yourself up for success, remove tempting processed foods, refined sugars, and unhealthy fats from your pantry and refrigerator. Stock up on nutrient-dense whole foods like vegetables, fruits, lean proteins, nuts, and seeds.

5. **Plan Your Meals**: Spend some time each week planning your meals and snacks to ensure you have nourishing options on hand. Aim for a balance of protein, healthy fats, and complex carbohydrates at each meal, and incorporate plenty of vegetables and fiber-rich foods.

6. **Start Slowly with Intermittent Fasting**: If you're new to intermittent fasting, start slowly by gradually extending your fasting window over time. Begin with a 12-hour fast

overnight and gradually increase to 14, 16, or even 18 hours if desired.

7. **Listen to Your Body**: Pay attention to how different foods make you feel and adjust your diet accordingly. If you notice any negative symptoms or reactions, such as bloating, fatigue, or mood swings, consider eliminating or reducing those foods from your diet.

8. **Stay Hydrated**: Proper hydration is essential for overall health and well-being. Aim to drink plenty of water throughout the day, and consider incorporating herbal teas and infused water for added flavor and hydration.

9. **Be Patient and Persistent**: Rome wasn't built in a day, and neither are lasting changes to your health and lifestyle. Be patient with yourself and trust the process, even if progress feels slow at times. Stay consistent with your dietary choices and lifestyle habits, and the results will come.

10. **Seek Support and Accountability**: Consider joining a community or support group of fellow Galveston Diet practitioners for encouragement, accountability, and inspiration. Having a supportive network can make all the difference on your journey to better health.

By following these steps and staying committed to your health goals, you can successfully embark on your Galveston Diet journey and experience the transformative benefits it has to offer. Remember, it's not just about what you eat, but how you nourish your body and prioritize your well-being.

CHAPTER TWO

Galveston Diet Basics

The Galveston Diet is built upon foundational principles that focus on optimizing macronutrient intake, understanding the role of hormones in weight loss and health, and balancing hormones through dietary strategies. In this section, we'll delve into these fundamental aspects to provide a comprehensive understanding of the Galveston Diet.

Understanding Macronutrients: Proteins, Carbs, and Fats

Macronutrients are the three primary components of food that provide energy and essential nutrients to the body: proteins, carbohydrates, and fats. Understanding how to balance these macronutrients is crucial for optimizing health and achieving weight loss goals on the Galveston Diet.

1. **Proteins**: Proteins are the building blocks of the body, essential for tissue repair, muscle growth, and hormone production. Incorporating an adequate amount of protein into your diet is key for maintaining muscle mass, supporting metabolism, and promoting satiety. Good sources of protein include lean meats, poultry, fish, eggs, dairy products, legumes, and tofu.

2. **Carbohydrates**: Carbohydrates are the body's primary source of energy, but not all carbs are created equal. The Galveston Diet emphasizes complex carbohydrates, such as whole grains, vegetables, fruits, and legumes, which are rich in fiber and nutrients and promote stable blood sugar levels.

It advises against or limits refined carbohydrates and sugars, which can lead to blood sugar spikes and inflammation.

3. **Fats**: Dietary fats are essential for hormone production, brain function, and nutrient absorption. The Galveston Diet encourages the consumption of healthy fats, including monounsaturated and polyunsaturated fats found in foods like avocados, nuts, seeds, olive oil, and fatty fish. These fats can help reduce inflammation and support hormonal balance.

Balancing macronutrients on the Galveston Diet involves incorporating a variety of whole foods rich in protein, complex carbohydrates, and healthy fats into your meals and snacks. This balanced approach helps stabilize blood sugar levels, promote satiety, and support overall health and well-being.

The Role of Hormones in Weight Loss and Health

Hormones play a significant role in regulating metabolism, appetite, energy expenditure, and fat storage, making them crucial factors in weight loss and overall health. Understanding how hormones influence these processes is key to achieving success on the Galveston Diet.

1. **Insulin**: Insulin is a hormone produced by the pancreas that regulates blood sugar levels by facilitating the uptake of

glucose into cells. High insulin levels, often caused by excessive carbohydrate intake or insulin resistance, can promote fat storage and inhibit fat burning. The Galveston Diet aims to regulate insulin levels through balanced macronutrient intake and mindful carbohydrate consumption.

2. **Leptin and Ghrelin**: Leptin and ghrelin are hormones involved in appetite regulation. Leptin, produced by fat cells, signals satiety to the brain, while ghrelin, produced by the stomach, stimulates hunger. Imbalances in these hormones can lead to overeating and weight gain. The Galveston Diet promotes satiety and hunger control through nutrient-dense foods and strategic meal timing.

3. **Estrogen and Progesterone**: Estrogen and progesterone are sex hormones that play a role in metabolism, fat distribution, and energy balance. During perimenopause and menopause, fluctuations in estrogen and progesterone levels can contribute to weight gain, particularly around the abdomen. The Galveston Diet aims to support hormonal balance through dietary strategies that minimize inflammation and stabilize blood sugar levels.

4. **Cortisol**: Cortisol is known as the stress hormone and is released in response to stress and low blood sugar levels. Chronically elevated cortisol levels can lead to abdominal fat

deposition, insulin resistance, and metabolic dysfunction. The Galveston Diet promotes stress management techniques, such as meditation, mindfulness, and adequate sleep, to help regulate cortisol levels and support overall health.

By addressing hormonal imbalances through dietary and lifestyle interventions, the Galveston Diet aims to optimize metabolism, promote fat loss, and improve overall health and well-being.

How to Balance Hormones with the Galveston Diet

Balancing hormones is a central focus of the Galveston Diet, as hormonal imbalances can contribute to weight gain, metabolic dysfunction, and other health issues. Here are some strategies for balancing hormones through the Galveston Diet:

1. **Eat Balanced Meals**: Focus on meals that contain a balance of protein, healthy fats, and complex carbohydrates. This balanced macronutrient intake helps stabilize blood sugar levels and regulate insulin secretion, supporting hormonal balance.

2. **Choose Hormone-Supportive Foods**: Incorporate foods rich in nutrients that support hormone production and metabolism, such as leafy greens, cruciferous vegetables, fatty fish, avocados, nuts, seeds, and berries. These foods

provide essential vitamins, minerals, antioxidants, and omega-3 fatty acids that promote hormonal health.

3. **Limit Sugar and Processed Foods**: Minimize consumption of refined carbohydrates, sugars, and processed foods, which can spike blood sugar levels, promote inflammation, and disrupt hormonal balance. Instead, opt for whole, unprocessed foods that nourish the body and support metabolic health.

4. **Practice Intermittent Fasting**: Intermittent fasting can help regulate insulin levels, improve insulin sensitivity, and promote fat burning. Experiment with different fasting protocols, such as the 16:8 method or alternate-day fasting, to find what works best for your body and lifestyle.

5. **Manage Stress**: Chronic stress can disrupt hormone balance and contribute to weight gain and metabolic dysfunction. Incorporate stress management techniques into your daily routine, such as meditation, deep breathing exercises, yoga, or spending time in nature.

6. **Get Adequate Sleep**: Prioritize quality sleep, as insufficient sleep can disrupt hormone production, increase hunger and cravings, and impair metabolism. Aim for 7-9 hours of restful sleep per night and establish a relaxing bedtime routine to promote optimal sleep quality.

7. **Stay Hydrated**: Hydration is essential for hormone production, metabolism, and overall health. Drink plenty of water throughout the day to support hydration levels and facilitate metabolic processes.

8. **Seek Professional Guidance**: If you're struggling with hormone imbalances or weight management issues, consider consulting with a healthcare provider or registered dietitian who specializes in hormonal health. They can offer personalized guidance and support to help you achieve your health goals.

By implementing these strategies and adopting a hormone-balancing approach to eating and lifestyle habits, you can support optimal hormone function, improve metabolic health, and achieve lasting weight loss and overall well-being with the Galveston Diet.

CHAPTER THREE

Setting Up Your Kitchen for Success

Setting up your kitchen for success is an essential step in following any dietary plan, including the Galveston Diet. From having the right tools and equipment to stocking your pantry with the necessary staples and mastering smart grocery shopping, a well-prepared kitchen can make it easier to stay on track with your health and wellness goals. In this section, we'll explore how to set up your kitchen for success on the Galveston Diet.

Essential Tools and Equipment for Galveston Diet Beginners

Having the right tools and equipment in your kitchen can streamline meal preparation and make it easier to stick to the Galveston Diet. Here are some essential items to have on hand:

1. **Quality Knives**: Invest in a set of sharp, high-quality knives for slicing, dicing, and chopping fruits, vegetables, and proteins.

2. **Cutting Boards**: Use cutting boards made of wood or plastic to protect your countertops and prevent cross-contamination while preparing food.

3. **Cookware**: Stock your kitchen with basic cookware, including pots, pans, and baking sheets, made from materials such as stainless steel, cast iron, or ceramic.

4. **Food Processor or Blender**: A food processor or blender is useful for making sauces, smoothies, soups, and other recipes that require blending or pureeing ingredients.

5. **Measuring Cups and Spoons**: Accurate measurement is crucial for following recipes and portion control. Have a set of measuring cups and spoons for precise ingredient measurements.

6. **Digital Kitchen Scale**: A digital kitchen scale can be helpful for portion control and accurately measuring ingredients, especially when following recipes that list measurements by weight.

7. **Slow Cooker or Instant Pot**: These versatile kitchen appliances make it easy to prepare healthy meals with minimal effort, perfect for busy days or meal prep.

8. **Storage Containers**: Invest in a variety of storage containers for storing leftovers, prepped ingredients, and batch-cooked meals. Choose containers that are microwave-safe, dishwasher-safe, and freezer-safe for added convenience.

9. **Vegetable Spiralizer**: A vegetable spiralizer is a fun tool for turning vegetables like zucchini, carrots, and sweet potatoes into noodles or spirals, offering a low-carb alternative to traditional pasta.

10.   **Grill or Grill Pan**: Grilling is a healthy cooking method that adds flavor to meats, vegetables, and fish without the need for added fats or oils. A grill or grill pan allows you to enjoy grilled foods year-round, even indoors.

Having these essential tools and equipment in your kitchen can make meal preparation more efficient and enjoyable, helping you stay consistent with the Galveston Diet.

Stocking Your Pantry with Galveston Diet Staples

Stocking your pantry with Galveston Diet staples ensures you always have nourishing ingredients on hand to create healthy, balanced meals. Here are some staple items to keep in your pantry:

1. **Whole Grains**: Choose whole grains such as quinoa, brown rice, oats, barley, and farro for fiber-rich carbohydrate options that promote satiety and stabilize blood sugar levels.

2. **Legumes**: Stock up on canned or dried legumes like black beans, chickpeas, lentils, and kidney beans for plant-based protein, fiber, and essential nutrients.

3. **Healthy Oils**: Opt for heart-healthy oils like olive oil, avocado oil, coconut oil, and walnut oil for cooking, salad dressings, and flavoring dishes.

4. **Nuts and Seeds**: Keep a variety of nuts and seeds on hand for snacking, adding crunch to salads and yogurt, or incorporating into recipes. Almonds, walnuts, chia seeds, flaxseeds, and pumpkin seeds are excellent choices.

5. **Nut and Seed Butters**: Choose natural nut and seed butters made from just nuts or seeds without added sugars or oils. Peanut butter, almond butter, and tahini are versatile options for adding flavor and nutrition to meals and snacks.

6. **Canned Fish**: Stock your pantry with canned fish like salmon, tuna, and sardines for convenient sources of omega-3 fatty acids, protein, and minerals.

7. **Herbs and Spices**: Build a collection of herbs, spices, and seasonings to add flavor to your meals without relying on excess salt or sugar. Common options include garlic powder, onion powder, cumin, paprika, basil, oregano, and turmeric.

8. **Canned Tomatoes and Tomato Paste**: Canned tomatoes and tomato paste are pantry staples that add depth of flavor to sauces, soups, and stews.

9. **Coconut Milk**: Coconut milk is a versatile ingredient for adding creaminess to curries, soups, smoothies, and desserts. Opt for canned coconut milk without added sugars or preservatives.

10. **Low-Sodium Broth or Stock**: Keep low-sodium vegetable, chicken, or beef broth on hand for making soups, stews, and sauces.

By keeping these staple items in your pantry, you'll have the foundation for creating a wide variety of nutritious and delicious meals that align with the principles of the Galveston Diet.

Smart Grocery Shopping Tips for Beginners

Navigating the grocery store can be overwhelming, but with some smart shopping strategies, you can make healthier choices and stay on track with the Galveston Diet. Here are some tips for successful grocery shopping:

1. **Plan Ahead**: Before heading to the store, take some time to plan your meals for the week and make a shopping list based on your meal plan. This will help you avoid impulse purchases and ensure you have everything you need for healthy meals.

2. **Shop the Perimeter**: Stick to the perimeter of the grocery store where fresh produce, lean meats, dairy products, and whole foods are typically located. Avoid the inner aisles where processed and packaged foods are often found.

3. **Read Labels**: When selecting packaged foods, take the time to read labels and ingredients lists. Look for products with

minimal ingredients, no added sugars, and no artificial additives or preservatives.

4. **Choose Whole Foods**: Opt for whole, minimally processed foods whenever possible. Choose fresh fruits and vegetables, lean proteins, whole grains, and healthy fats over pre-packaged or convenience foods.

5. **Buy in Bulk**: Consider buying staple items like grains, legumes, nuts, and seeds in bulk to save money and reduce packaging waste. Be mindful of portion sizes to avoid overbuying perishable items.

6. **Focus on Seasonal Produce**: Choose fruits and vegetables that are in season for the freshest flavors and the best nutritional value. Seasonal produce is often more affordable and locally sourced.

7. **Compare Prices**: Compare prices between different brands and store options to find the best value for your money. Consider shopping at farmers' markets or discount grocers for budget-friendly options.

8. **Limit Processed Foods**: Minimize purchases of processed foods like sugary snacks, chips, and frozen meals, which are often high in unhealthy fats, sugars, and sodium. Instead, prioritize whole, nutrient-dense foods.

9. **Be Flexible**: Stay open to trying new foods and recipes to keep your meals interesting and varied. Experiment with different ingredients and cooking methods to discover what you enjoy.

10. **Stick to Your List**: Resist the temptation to stray from your shopping list and impulse buy items that don't align with your dietary goals. Focus on purchasing the items you need to support your health and well-being.

By following these smart grocery shopping tips, you can make healthier choices and stock your kitchen with the ingredients you need to succeed on the Galveston Diet. With careful planning and mindful shopping, you can set yourself up for success in achieving your health and wellness goals.

CHAPTER FOUR

Breakfast Essentials

Breakfast is often considered the most important meal of the day, and on the Galveston Diet, it's an opportunity to kickstart your metabolism, stabilize blood sugar levels, and fuel your body with nourishing foods. In this section, we'll explore essential breakfast ideas for beginners on the Galveston Diet, including quick and easy options, energizing smoothie recipes, and satisfying breakfast bowls.

Quick and Easy Galveston Diet Breakfast Ideas for Beginners

Starting your day with a nutritious breakfast doesn't have to be complicated or time-consuming. Here are some quick and easy breakfast ideas for beginners on the Galveston Diet:

1. **Greek Yogurt Parfait**: Layer Greek yogurt with fresh berries, nuts, and a drizzle of honey or a sprinkle of cinnamon for a protein-rich and satisfying breakfast option.

2. **Avocado Toast**: Top whole grain toast with mashed avocado, sliced tomatoes, and a sprinkle of sea salt and black pepper for a simple and delicious breakfast loaded with healthy fats and fiber.

3. **Egg Muffins**: Whip up a batch of egg muffins by combining beaten eggs with chopped vegetables, cheese, and cooked

lean protein like turkey sausage or diced ham. Pour the mixture into muffin tins and bake until set for a portable and protein-packed breakfast option.

4. **Overnight Oats**: Prepare overnight oats by combining rolled oats with Greek yogurt, milk or almond milk, chia seeds, and your choice of toppings such as berries, nuts, and nut butter. Let the mixture soak overnight in the refrigerator, and enjoy a ready-to-eat breakfast in the morning.

5. **Nut Butter Banana Wrap**: Spread your favorite nut butter on a whole grain tortilla, top with sliced banana, and sprinkle with cinnamon. Roll up the tortilla and enjoy a nutrient-dense and portable breakfast option.

6. **Chia Seed Pudding**: Mix chia seeds with milk or coconut milk, sweeten with a touch of honey or maple syrup, and let the mixture sit in the refrigerator overnight to thicken into a pudding-like consistency. Top with fresh fruit, nuts, and seeds for a satisfying breakfast treat.

7. **Vegetable Omelet**: Whip up a quick vegetable omelet by sautéing chopped vegetables like spinach, bell peppers, onions, and mushrooms in olive oil, then pouring beaten eggs over the vegetables and cooking until set. Serve with a side of whole grain toast for a balanced breakfast.

8. **Smoothie Bowl**: Blend together your favorite fruits, leafy greens, protein powder, and liquid of choice to create a thick and creamy smoothie base. Pour the smoothie into a bowl and top with granola, nuts, seeds, and additional fruit for added texture and flavor.

9. **Breakfast Tacos**: Fill whole grain tortillas with scrambled eggs, black beans, avocado slices, salsa, and a sprinkle of cheese for a savory and satisfying breakfast option.

10. **Whole Grain Pancakes**: Make a batch of whole grain pancakes using a mix of whole wheat flour, oats, and mashed banana for natural sweetness. Serve with Greek yogurt and fresh fruit for added protein and fiber.

These quick and easy breakfast ideas are perfect for beginners on the Galveston Diet and can be customized to suit your taste preferences and dietary needs.

Energizing Smoothie Recipes for Breakfast Beginners

Smoothies are a convenient and delicious way to pack a variety of nutrients into your breakfast routine. Here are some energizing smoothie recipes for beginners on the Galveston Diet:

1. **Green Goddess Smoothie**: Blend together spinach, kale, banana, Greek yogurt, almond milk, and a scoop of protein

powder for a nutrient-packed smoothie that's rich in vitamins, minerals, and antioxidants.

2. **Berry Blast Smoothie**: Combine mixed berries, banana, spinach, almond milk, and a tablespoon of chia seeds for a refreshing and antioxidant-rich smoothie that's perfect for jumpstarting your day.

3. **Tropical Paradise Smoothie**: Blend together pineapple, mango, coconut milk, Greek yogurt, and a splash of orange juice for a tropical-inspired smoothie that's bursting with flavor and energy-boosting nutrients.

4. **Chocolate Peanut Butter Smoothie**: Mix together cocoa powder, banana, peanut butter, Greek yogurt, almond milk, and a handful of spinach for a decadent and protein-rich smoothie that tastes like dessert.

5. **Coffee Protein Smoothie**: Brew a strong cup of coffee and let it cool, then blend it with banana, almond milk, protein powder, and a handful of ice for a caffeinated and protein-packed breakfast pick-me-up.

6. **Antioxidant Powerhouse Smoothie**: Combine acai berries, blueberries, strawberries, banana, spinach, almond milk, and a scoop of protein powder for a vibrant and antioxidant-rich smoothie that's as nutritious as it is delicious.

7. **Minty Green Smoothie**: Blend together spinach, banana, fresh mint leaves, Greek yogurt, almond milk, and a squeeze of lime juice for a refreshing and invigorating smoothie that's perfect for starting your day on a fresh note.

8. **Peaches and Cream Smoothie**: Mix together ripe peaches, banana, Greek yogurt, almond milk, and a splash of vanilla extract for a creamy and satisfying smoothie that tastes like summer in a glass.

9. **Detox Green Smoothie**: Combine cucumber, celery, parsley, lemon juice, ginger, pineapple, spinach, and coconut water for a cleansing and refreshing smoothie that's packed with detoxifying nutrients.

10. **Banana Almond Smoothie**: Blend together banana, almond butter, Greek yogurt, almond milk, and a sprinkle of cinnamon for a creamy and protein-rich smoothie that will keep you satisfied all morning long.

These energizing smoothie recipes are perfect for beginners on the Galveston Diet and can be customized with your favorite fruits, vegetables, and add-ins to suit your taste preferences and nutritional needs.

Simple and Satisfying Breakfast Bowls for Beginners

Breakfast bowls offer a customizable and satisfying way to enjoy a nutritious morning meal. Here are some simple and satisfying breakfast bowl ideas for beginners on the Galveston Diet:

1. **Acai Bowl**: Top a base of acai puree or blended frozen acai berries with granola, sliced banana, berries, coconut flakes, and a drizzle of honey for a nourishing and antioxidant-rich breakfast bowl.

2. **Greek Yogurt Bowl**: Start with a base of Greek yogurt and top with sliced fruit, nuts, seeds, and a sprinkle of granola or muesli for a protein-packed and satisfying breakfast option.

3. **Quinoa Breakfast Bowl**: Cook quinoa according to package instructions and top with sautéed spinach, cherry tomatoes, avocado slices, a poached egg, and a drizzle of tahini or hot sauce for a hearty and nutrient-dense breakfast bowl.

4. **Chia Seed Pudding Bowl**: Spoon chia seed pudding into a bowl and top with sliced banana, berries, nuts, seeds, and a drizzle of almond butter or maple syrup for a creamy and satisfying breakfast treat.

5. **Oatmeal Breakfast Bowl**: Cook rolled oats with almond milk or water and top with sliced fruit, nuts, seeds, and a sprinkle

of cinnamon or nutmeg for a warm and comforting breakfast bowl that's perfect for chilly mornings.

6. **Smoothie Bowl**: Pour your favorite smoothie into a bowl and top with granola, sliced fruit, nuts, seeds, and a drizzle of honey or nut butter for a thick and creamy breakfast bowl that's as delicious as it is nutritious.

7. **Egg and Vegetable Breakfast Bowl**: Sauté mixed vegetables like bell peppers, onions, mushrooms, and spinach in olive oil and top with scrambled eggs, avocado slices, and a sprinkle of cheese for a savory and satisfying breakfast option.

8. **Tofu Scramble Bowl**: Crumble firm tofu and sauté with mixed vegetables, spices, and seasonings until heated through. Serve over cooked quinoa or brown rice and top with avocado slices and salsa for a protein-rich and plant-based breakfast bowl.

9. **Mediterranean Breakfast Bowl**: Combine cooked farro or barley with cherry tomatoes, cucumber slices, Kalamata olives, feta cheese, and a drizzle of olive oil and balsamic vinegar for a Mediterranean-inspired breakfast bowl that's full of flavor and nutrition.

10. **Coconut Chia Breakfast Bowl**: Mix together chia seeds, coconut milk, shredded coconut, and a touch of honey or maple syrup and let the mixture sit in the refrigerator

overnight to thicken. Top with sliced mango, pineapple, and kiwi for a tropical-inspired breakfast bowl that's perfect for summer mornings.

These simple and satisfying breakfast bowl ideas are perfect for beginners on the Galveston Diet and can be customized with your favorite ingredients to create delicious and nutritious morning meals.

CHAPTER FIVE

Lunchtime Favorites

Lunch is an important opportunity to refuel your body and nourish yourself with nutritious foods, especially when following the Galveston Diet. In this section, we'll explore some lunchtime favorites perfect for beginners on the Galveston Diet, including beginner-friendly salad recipes, wholesome soup and stew recipes, and easy-to-make sandwiches and wraps.

Beginner-Friendly Salad Recipes for Galveston Dieters

Salads are versatile, nutrient-rich meals that can be customized to suit your taste preferences and dietary needs. Here are some beginner-friendly salad recipes for Galveston dieters:

1. **Classic Garden Salad**: Combine mixed greens, cherry tomatoes, cucumber slices, shredded carrots, and bell pepper strips in a large bowl. Top with a sprinkle of feta cheese, sunflower seeds, and a drizzle of balsamic vinaigrette for a simple and refreshing salad option.

2. **Greek Salad**: Toss together romaine lettuce, sliced cucumber, cherry tomatoes, Kalamata olives, red onion slices, and crumbled feta cheese in a bowl. Dress with a mixture of olive oil, lemon juice, garlic, oregano, salt, and pepper for a flavorful and satisfying Greek-inspired salad.

3. **Chicken Caesar Salad**: Top chopped romaine lettuce with grilled chicken breast slices, cherry tomatoes, shaved Parmesan cheese, and whole grain croutons. Drizzle with Caesar dressing and toss to coat for a protein-rich and satisfying salad option.

4. **Quinoa Veggie Salad**: Combine cooked quinoa with diced bell peppers, cherry tomatoes, cucumber slices, shredded carrots, and chopped parsley in a bowl. Dress with a lemon-tahini dressing made from tahini, lemon juice, garlic, salt, and pepper for a hearty and nutritious salad option.

5. **Taco Salad**: Layer chopped romaine lettuce with seasoned ground turkey or beef, black beans, diced avocado, cherry tomatoes, shredded cheese, and crushed tortilla chips in a bowl. Top with salsa and Greek yogurt or sour cream for a flavorful and satisfying taco-inspired salad.

6. **Asian Chicken Salad**: Toss together shredded cabbage, carrots, bell peppers, sliced green onions, and chopped cilantro in a bowl. Top with grilled chicken breast slices and drizzle with a homemade sesame-ginger dressing made from sesame oil, rice vinegar, soy sauce, honey, ginger, and garlic for an Asian-inspired salad option.

7. **Mediterranean Quinoa Salad**: Combine cooked quinoa with diced cucumber, cherry tomatoes, Kalamata olives, red onion slices, crumbled feta cheese, and chopped parsley in a

bowl. Dress with a mixture of olive oil, lemon juice, garlic, oregano, salt, and pepper for a flavorful and satisfying Mediterranean-inspired salad.

8. **Caprese Salad**: Arrange sliced tomatoes, fresh mozzarella cheese slices, and fresh basil leaves on a platter. Drizzle with balsamic glaze and extra virgin olive oil, and sprinkle with sea salt and black pepper for a simple and elegant Italian-inspired salad option.

9. **Cobb Salad**: Arrange chopped romaine lettuce in a bowl and top with rows of cooked chopped chicken breast, hard-boiled egg slices, crumbled bacon, avocado slices, cherry tomatoes, and crumbled blue cheese. Serve with a side of ranch dressing for a classic and hearty salad option.

10. **Spinach and Strawberry Salad**: Combine baby spinach leaves with sliced strawberries, crumbled goat cheese, and toasted almonds in a bowl. Dress with a balsamic vinaigrette made from balsamic vinegar, olive oil, honey, Dijon mustard, salt, and pepper for a sweet and savory salad option.

These beginner-friendly salad recipes are perfect for Galveston dieters and can be enjoyed as a satisfying and nutritious lunch option.

Wholesome Soup and Stew Recipes for Beginners

Soup and stew are comforting and nourishing meals that can be easily customized to suit your taste preferences and dietary needs. Here are some wholesome soup and stew recipes for beginners:

1. **Vegetable Soup**: In a large pot, combine chopped vegetables such as carrots, celery, onions, bell peppers, and zucchini with vegetable broth, diced tomatoes, and cooked beans or lentils. Season with herbs and spices like garlic, thyme, rosemary, and bay leaves, and simmer until vegetables are tender for a hearty and nutritious vegetable soup option.

2. **Chicken Noodle Soup**: In a large pot, combine diced cooked chicken breast, chopped carrots, celery, onions, and garlic with chicken broth and cooked whole grain pasta. Season with herbs like parsley, thyme, and bay leaves, and simmer until vegetables are tender for a comforting and classic chicken noodle soup option.

3. **Minestrone Soup**: In a large pot, combine diced onions, carrots, celery, zucchini, and green beans with vegetable broth, diced tomatoes, cooked beans or lentils, and whole grain pasta. Season with Italian herbs like basil, oregano, and thyme, and simmer until vegetables are tender for a hearty and flavorful minestrone soup option.

4. **Black Bean Soup**: In a large pot, combine diced onions, bell peppers, and garlic with vegetable broth, canned black beans, diced tomatoes, and corn kernels. Season with cumin, chili powder, and smoked paprika, and simmer until flavors are blended for a spicy and satisfying black bean soup option.

5. **Tomato Basil Soup**: In a large pot, combine diced onions, carrots, and celery with vegetable broth, canned diced tomatoes, and fresh basil leaves. Simmer until vegetables are tender, then puree the soup until smooth using an immersion blender or countertop blender for a creamy and comforting tomato basil soup option.

6. **Butternut Squash Soup**: In a large pot, combine diced butternut squash, onions, carrots, and apples with vegetable broth and coconut milk. Season with warming spices like cinnamon, nutmeg, and ginger, and simmer until vegetables are tender for a creamy and comforting butternut squash soup option.

7. **Lentil Soup**: In a large pot, combine diced onions, carrots, celery, and garlic with vegetable broth, dried lentils, canned diced tomatoes, and spinach. Season with herbs like thyme, rosemary, and bay leaves, and simmer until lentils are tender for a hearty and nutritious lentil soup option.

8. **Turkey Chili**: In a large pot, combine lean ground turkey, diced onions, bell peppers, and garlic with canned kidney beans, diced tomatoes, tomato sauce, and chili powder. Simmer until flavors are blended and chili is thickened for a spicy and satisfying turkey chili option.

9. **Potato Leek Soup**: In a large pot, combine diced potatoes, leeks, onions, and garlic with vegetable broth and a splash of cream or coconut milk. Simmer until vegetables are tender, then puree the soup until smooth for a creamy and comforting potato leek soup option.

10.   **Beef and Vegetable Stew**: In a large pot or slow cooker, combine cubed beef stew meat with diced onions, carrots, celery, potatoes, and garlic. Add beef broth, diced tomatoes, and herbs like thyme, rosemary, and bay leaves. Simmer until beef is tender and vegetables are cooked through for a hearty and satisfying beef and vegetable stew option.

These wholesome soup and stew recipes are perfect for beginners on the Galveston Diet and can be enjoyed as a comforting and nutritious lunch option.

Easy-to-Make Sandwiches and Wraps for Beginners

Sandwiches and wraps are convenient and portable meal options that can be customized with your favorite ingredients and flavors.

Here are some easy-to-make sandwich and wrap recipes for beginners:

1. **Turkey and Avocado Sandwich**: Layer sliced turkey breast, mashed avocado, lettuce, tomato, and sliced cucumber on whole grain bread. Add a dollop of Greek yogurt or mustard for extra flavor, and enjoy a satisfying and protein-rich sandwich option.

2. **Caprese Sandwich**: Stack sliced tomatoes, fresh mozzarella cheese, and basil leaves on whole grain bread. Drizzle with balsamic glaze and extra virgin olive oil, and season with sea salt and black pepper for a simple and elegant Italian-inspired sandwich option.

3. **Grilled Chicken Caesar Wrap**: Fill a whole grain wrap with grilled chicken breast slices, romaine lettuce, Parmesan cheese, and Caesar dressing. Roll up the wrap and enjoy a classic and protein-packed lunch option.

4. **Veggie Hummus Wrap**: Spread hummus on a whole grain wrap and layer with sliced cucumber, bell peppers, carrots, lettuce, and avocado. Roll up the wrap and enjoy a flavorful and nutrient-rich lunch option.

5. **Tuna Salad Sandwich**: Mix canned tuna with Greek yogurt or mayonnaise, diced celery, red onion, and dill pickle relish. Spread the tuna salad on whole grain bread and top with

lettuce and tomato for a classic and protein-rich sandwich option.

6. **BLT Wrap**: Fill a whole grain wrap with cooked bacon slices, lettuce, tomato, and sliced avocado. Drizzle with Greek yogurt or mayonnaise and roll up the wrap for a classic and satisfying lunch option.

7. **Egg Salad Sandwich**: Mash hard-boiled eggs with Greek yogurt or mayonnaise, Dijon mustard, and chopped chives. Spread the egg salad on whole grain bread and top with lettuce and tomato for a protein-rich and satisfying sandwich option.

8. **Mediterranean Veggie Wrap**: Fill a whole grain wrap with roasted vegetables like eggplant, zucchini, bell peppers, and red onion. Add crumbled feta cheese, Kalamata olives, and hummus, and roll up the wrap for a flavorful and nutrient-rich lunch option.

9. **Turkey and Cranberry Wrap**: Spread cream cheese on a whole grain wrap and layer with sliced turkey breast, cranberry sauce, and spinach leaves. Roll up the wrap and enjoy a festive and flavorful lunch option.

10. **Quinoa and Black Bean Wrap**: Combine cooked quinoa with black beans, diced tomatoes, corn kernels, chopped cilantro, and lime juice. Spread the quinoa mixture on a

whole grain wrap and top with shredded cheese and avocado slices for a hearty and nutritious lunch option.

These easy-to-make sandwich and wrap recipes are perfect for beginners on the Galveston Diet and can be customized with your favorite ingredients and flavors for a delicious and satisfying lunch option.

CHAPTER SIX

Snacks for Success

Snacking can be an important part of a balanced diet, providing energy between meals and helping to curb hunger and prevent overeating. For beginners on the Galveston Diet, choosing nutritious snacks that align with the program's principles is key to staying on track with health and wellness goals. In this section, we'll explore a variety of snacks perfect for success on the Galveston Diet, including healthy snack ideas, quick and simple snack recipes, and portable snacks for on-the-go beginners.

Healthy Snack Ideas for Galveston Diet Beginners

Choosing healthy snacks that are nutrient-dense and satisfying is essential for success on the Galveston Diet. Here are some healthy snack ideas for beginners:

1. **Fresh Fruit**: Enjoy whole fruits like apples, bananas, berries, oranges, and grapes for a naturally sweet and refreshing snack option that's rich in vitamins, minerals, and fiber.

2. **Vegetable Sticks and Hummus**: Dip crunchy vegetable sticks such as carrots, celery, bell peppers, and cucumber into creamy hummus for a satisfying and nutrient-rich snack option.

3. **Greek Yogurt and Berries**: Pair Greek yogurt with fresh berries like strawberries, blueberries, or raspberries for a protein-rich and antioxidant-packed snack that's both creamy and satisfying.

4. **Nut Butter and Apple Slices**: Spread your favorite nut butter like almond butter or peanut butter on apple slices for a crunchy and satisfying snack option that combines healthy fats, protein, and fiber.

5. **Hard-Boiled Eggs**: Enjoy hard-boiled eggs as a portable and protein-rich snack option that's easy to prepare and perfect for on-the-go snacking.

6. **Mixed Nuts and Seeds**: Create your own trail mix by combining a variety of nuts and seeds such as almonds, walnuts, pumpkin seeds, and sunflower seeds for a crunchy and nutrient-rich snack option.

7. **Cheese and Whole Grain Crackers**: Pair sliced cheese with whole grain crackers for a satisfying and balanced snack option that provides a mix of protein, carbohydrates, and healthy fats.

8. **Cottage Cheese and Pineapple**: Combine cottage cheese with diced pineapple for a creamy and refreshing snack option that's high in protein and packed with tropical flavor.

9. **Roasted Chickpeas**: Season cooked chickpeas with spices like paprika, cumin, and garlic powder, then roast in the oven until crispy for a crunchy and protein-rich snack option.

10. **Yogurt Parfait**: Layer Greek yogurt with granola, fresh fruit, and a drizzle of honey for a satisfying and customizable snack option that's perfect for any time of day.

These healthy snack ideas are perfect for beginners on the Galveston Diet and can help support energy levels, curb hunger, and promote overall well-being.

Quick and Simple Snack Recipes for Beginners

Preparing homemade snacks can be a great way to ensure you're getting wholesome ingredients and avoiding added sugars and preservatives. Here are some quick and simple snack recipes for beginners:

1. **Energy Bites**: Combine rolled oats, nut butter, honey, and mix-ins like chocolate chips, dried fruit, or nuts in a bowl. Roll the mixture into bite-sized balls and refrigerate until firm for a portable and energy-boosting snack option.

2. **Vegetable Sushi Rolls**: Spread cooked quinoa or brown rice onto nori sheets, then layer with sliced vegetables like cucumber, avocado, and bell peppers. Roll up the sushi rolls tightly and slice into bite-sized pieces for a nutritious and satisfying snack option.

3. **Stuffed Bell Peppers**: Slice bell peppers in half and remove the seeds and membranes. Fill the pepper halves with a mixture of cottage cheese, diced tomatoes, and herbs like basil and oregano. Bake until peppers are tender for a creamy and flavorful snack option.

4. **Homemade Trail Mix**: Combine a variety of nuts, seeds, dried fruit, and dark chocolate chips in a bowl. Mix well and portion into individual servings for a convenient and customizable snack option.

5. **Avocado Toast with Egg**: Mash avocado onto whole grain toast and top with a cooked egg for a protein-rich and satisfying snack option that's perfect for any time of day.

6. **Frozen Yogurt Bark**: Spread Greek yogurt onto a baking sheet lined with parchment paper, then sprinkle with granola, berries, and a drizzle of honey. Freeze until firm, then break into pieces for a refreshing and nutritious snack option.

7. **Hummus and Veggie Pinwheels**: Spread hummus onto a whole grain tortilla, then layer with sliced vegetables like cucumber, bell peppers, and carrots. Roll up the tortilla tightly and slice into bite-sized pinwheels for a flavorful and portable snack option.

8. **Turkey and Cheese Roll-Ups**: Lay a slice of deli turkey on a flat surface, then top with a slice of cheese and a smear of mustard or hummus. Roll up tightly and slice into bite-sized pieces for a protein-rich and satisfying snack option.

9. **Fruit and Yogurt Popsicles**: Blend together Greek yogurt with mixed berries or tropical fruit, then pour into popsicle molds and freeze until firm for a refreshing and healthy snack option that's perfect for hot summer days.

10. **Quinoa Salad Cups**: Mix cooked quinoa with diced vegetables, herbs, and a squeeze of lemon juice. Spoon the quinoa salad into lettuce cups or halved bell peppers for a light and nutritious snack option.

These quick and simple snack recipes are perfect for beginners on the Galveston Diet and can be made ahead of time for easy grab-and-go snacking.

Portable Snacks for On-the-Go Beginners

When you're on the go, having portable snacks on hand can help you stay fueled and satisfied throughout the day. Here are some portable snacks perfect for beginners on the Galveston Diet:

1. **Apple Slices with Nut Butter**: Pack apple slices and single-serve packets of nut butter for a portable and satisfying snack option that combines natural sweetness with healthy fats and protein.

2. **String Cheese and Grapes**: Pair string cheese with grapes for a convenient and portable snack option that provides a mix of protein, calcium, and natural sweetness.

3. **Trail Mix Packets**: Portion homemade or store-bought trail mix into individual snack-sized bags for a convenient and customizable snack option that's perfect for on-the-go snacking.

4. **Greek Yogurt Cups**: Choose single-serve cups of Greek yogurt and top with granola or mixed berries for a protein-rich and portable snack option that's perfect for any time of day.

5. **Rice Cake with Avocado**: Spread mashed avocado onto rice cakes and sprinkle with sea salt and black pepper for a crunchy and satisfying snack option that's perfect for on-the-go snacking.

6. **Roasted Chickpea Snack Packs**: Portion roasted chickpeas into individual snack-sized bags for a crunchy and protein-rich snack option that's perfect for on-the-go snacking.

7. **Hard-Boiled Egg Packs**: Pack hard-boiled eggs into individual snack containers with a sprinkle of salt and pepper for a portable and protein-rich snack option that's perfect for on-the-go snacking.

8. **Vegetable and Hummus Cups**: Pack sliced vegetables like carrots, cucumber, and bell peppers into individual snack containers with a side of hummus for a crunchy and satisfying snack option that's perfect for on-the-go snacking.

9. **Nut and Seed Bars**: Choose store-bought or homemade nut and seed bars that are high in protein and fiber for a convenient and portable snack option that's perfect for on-the-go snacking.

10. **Dried Fruit Packs**: Portion dried fruit like apricots, figs, or mango into individual snack-sized bags for a naturally sweet and satisfying snack option that's perfect for on-the-go snacking.

These portable snacks are perfect for beginners on the Galveston Diet and can be enjoyed anytime, anywhere to help you stay fueled and satisfied throughout the day.

Conclusion

Snacking plays an important role in supporting energy levels, curbing hunger, and promoting overall well-being, especially for beginners on the Galveston Diet. By choosing nutritious snacks that align with the program's principles, such as fresh fruits and vegetables, lean proteins, and healthy fats, you can stay on track with your health and wellness goals. Whether you're looking for healthy snack ideas, quick and simple snack recipes, or portable snacks for on-the-go convenience, the options outlined in this section provide a variety of delicious and satisfying choices to support success on the Galveston Diet.

CHAPTER SEVEN

Dinner Made Easy

Dinner is often the main meal of the day, and it's important for it to be both satisfying and aligned with the principles of the Galveston Diet. In this section, we'll explore various dinner options that are easy to prepare, delicious, and perfect for beginners on the Galveston Diet.

Beginner-Friendly One-Pot Meals for Galveston Dieters

One-pot meals are a lifesaver for busy individuals who want a delicious dinner without spending hours in the kitchen or creating a mountain of dishes to wash afterward. Here are some beginner-friendly one-pot meal ideas that are perfect for Galveston dieters:

1. **Quinoa Vegetable Stir-Fry**: Cook quinoa according to package instructions. In a large skillet, sauté mixed vegetables such as bell peppers, broccoli, carrots, and snap peas until tender-crisp. Add cooked quinoa to the skillet and toss with soy sauce, garlic, and ginger for a flavorful and nutritious stir-fry.

2. **Chicken and Vegetable Skillet**: Season boneless, skinless chicken breasts with your favorite herbs and spices. In a large skillet, brown the chicken on both sides, then add chopped vegetables such as zucchini, bell peppers, and

onions to the skillet. Cover and cook until the chicken is cooked through and the vegetables are tender for a simple and satisfying meal.

3. **Shrimp and Quinoa Paella**: In a large skillet, sauté diced onions, bell peppers, and garlic until softened. Add uncooked quinoa, diced tomatoes, vegetable broth, and saffron (if available) to the skillet and bring to a simmer. Add shrimp and peas to the skillet and cook until the shrimp are pink and cooked through for a flavorful and protein-rich paella.

4. **Vegetarian Chili**: In a large pot, sauté diced onions, bell peppers, and garlic until softened. Add canned diced tomatoes, cooked beans (such as black beans, kidney beans, and chickpeas), vegetable broth, chili powder, cumin, and paprika to the pot. Simmer for 20-30 minutes until the flavors meld together for a hearty and comforting chili.

5. **Salmon and Vegetable Foil Packets**: Place salmon fillets on individual sheets of aluminum foil. Top with sliced vegetables such as zucchini, cherry tomatoes, and asparagus. Drizzle with olive oil, lemon juice, and your favorite herbs and spices. Seal the foil packets and bake in the oven until the salmon is cooked through and the vegetables are tender for a quick and flavorful meal.

6. **Turkey and Sweet Potato Hash**: In a large skillet, brown ground turkey with diced sweet potatoes, onions, and bell

peppers until the turkey is cooked through and the sweet potatoes are tender. Season with smoked paprika, cumin, and chili powder for a satisfying and nutritious hash.

7. **Lentil and Vegetable Soup**: In a large pot, sauté diced onions, carrots, and celery until softened. Add dried lentils, canned diced tomatoes, vegetable broth, and your favorite herbs and spices to the pot. Simmer for 20-30 minutes until the lentils are tender for a comforting and protein-rich soup.

8. **Beef and Broccoli Stir-Fry**: In a large skillet, brown thinly sliced beef strips with minced garlic and ginger until cooked through. Add broccoli florets and sliced bell peppers to the skillet and cook until tender-crisp. Toss with soy sauce, rice vinegar, and sesame oil for a flavorful and satisfying stir-fry.

9. **Spaghetti Squash with Turkey Bolognese**: Roast spaghetti squash halves in the oven until tender. Meanwhile, sauté ground turkey with diced onions, carrots, and garlic until browned. Add canned diced tomatoes, tomato paste, and Italian herbs to the skillet and simmer until the flavors meld together. Serve the turkey Bolognese over the roasted spaghetti squash for a lighter and healthier alternative to traditional pasta.

10. **Vegetable and Bean Stew**: In a large pot, sauté diced onions, carrots, and celery until softened. Add diced potatoes, canned diced tomatoes, vegetable broth, cooked

beans (such as cannellini beans or kidney beans), and your favorite herbs and spices to the pot. Simmer until the vegetables are tender and the flavors are well combined for a hearty and nutritious stew.

These beginner-friendly one-pot meals are perfect for Galveston dieters who want a quick, easy, and satisfying dinner option without sacrificing flavor or nutrition.

Delicious and Nutritious Seafood Recipes for Beginners

Seafood is not only delicious but also packed with essential nutrients such as omega-3 fatty acids, protein, vitamins, and minerals. Here are some delicious and nutritious seafood recipes that are perfect for beginners:

1. **Grilled Lemon Herb Salmon**: Marinate salmon fillets in a mixture of lemon juice, olive oil, minced garlic, and chopped fresh herbs such as parsley, dill, and thyme. Grill the salmon fillets until cooked through and flaky for a flavorful and nutritious meal.

2. **Baked Cod with Herbed Bread Crumbs**: Season cod fillets with salt, pepper, and lemon zest. Top with a mixture of whole grain breadcrumbs, chopped fresh herbs, and grated Parmesan cheese. Bake in the oven until the fish is cooked

through and the breadcrumbs are golden brown for a crispy
and delicious dish.

3. **Shrimp and Vegetable Stir-Fry**: In a large skillet, sauté diced
onions, bell peppers, and snap peas until tender-crisp. Add
peeled and deveined shrimp to the skillet and cook until pink
and cooked through. Toss with soy sauce, ginger, and garlic
for a quick and flavorful stir-fry.

4. **Tuna Salad Lettuce Wraps**: Mix canned tuna with Greek
yogurt, diced celery, red onion, and chopped pickles. Season
with salt, pepper, and lemon juice to taste. Spoon the tuna
salad into large lettuce leaves and roll them up for a light
and refreshing meal.

5. **Salmon and Asparagus Sheet Pan Dinner**: Place salmon
fillets and asparagus spears on a sheet pan. Drizzle with olive
oil and season with salt, pepper, and lemon zest. Roast in the
oven until the salmon is cooked through and the asparagus is
tender for an easy and nutritious dinner.

6. **Shrimp and Avocado Salad**: Toss cooked shrimp with diced
avocado, cherry tomatoes, cucumber, and mixed greens in a
large bowl. Drizzle with a simple vinaigrette made from olive
oil, lemon juice, Dijon mustard, and honey for a refreshing
and protein-rich salad option.

7. **Lemon Garlic Butter Scallops**: Sear sea scallops in a hot skillet with melted butter, minced garlic, and lemon zest until golden brown and caramelized on the outside and cooked through on the inside. Serve with a squeeze of lemon juice and chopped fresh parsley for a luxurious and flavorful dish.

8. **Tilapia Fish Tacos**: Season tilapia fillets with your favorite taco seasoning and grill or pan-sear until cooked through. Fill corn tortillas with the cooked tilapia, shredded cabbage or lettuce, diced tomatoes, avocado slices, and a dollop of Greek yogurt or sour cream for a delicious and satisfying taco option.

9. **Crab Cakes with Remoulade Sauce**: Mix lump crab meat with breadcrumbs, chopped green onions, minced bell peppers, and Old Bay seasoning. Form the mixture into patties and pan-fry until golden brown and crispy on the outside and cooked through on the inside. Serve with homemade remoulade sauce for a flavorful and indulgent meal.

10. **Shrimp and Quinoa Salad**: Cook quinoa according to package instructions and let cool. Toss cooked quinoa with cooked shrimp, diced cucumbers, cherry tomatoes, chopped fresh herbs, and a simple vinaigrette dressing for a light and protein-rich salad option.

These delicious and nutritious seafood recipes are perfect for beginners on the Galveston Diet who want to incorporate more seafood into their meals for its health benefits and delicious flavor.

Comforting Chicken and Turkey Dishes for Beginners

Chicken and turkey are versatile proteins that can be used in a wide variety of dishes, from comforting casseroles to flavorful stir-fries. Here are some comforting chicken and turkey dishes that are perfect for beginners:

1. **Baked Lemon Garlic Chicken**: Marinate chicken breasts in a mixture of lemon juice, olive oil, minced garlic, and dried herbs such as oregano, thyme, and rosemary. Bake in the oven until the chicken is cooked through and golden brown for a flavorful and aromatic dish.

2. **Turkey and Vegetable Skillet**: Brown ground turkey in a large skillet with diced onions, carrots, and celery until cooked through. Add diced potatoes, frozen peas, and your favorite herbs and spices to the skillet and cook until the vegetables are tender for a simple and comforting one-pan meal.

3. **Chicken and Broccoli Stir-Fry**: Thinly slice chicken breast and stir-fry in a hot skillet with minced garlic and ginger until

cooked through. Add broccoli florets and sliced bell peppers to the skillet and cook until tender-crisp. Toss with soy sauce and sesame oil for a quick and flavorful stir-fry.

4. **Turkey and Spinach Stuffed Peppers**: Cook ground turkey with diced onions, garlic, and spinach until browned. Season with Italian herbs and spices, then stuff the mixture into halved bell peppers. Bake until the peppers are tender and the filling is cooked through for a nutritious and filling meal.

5. **Chicken and Vegetable Soup**: In a large pot, sauté diced onions, carrots, and celery until softened. Add diced chicken breast, canned diced tomatoes, chicken broth, and your favorite herbs and spices to the pot. Simmer until the chicken is cooked through and the flavors meld together for a comforting and hearty soup option.

6. **Turkey Meatballs with Marinara Sauce**: Mix ground turkey with breadcrumbs, minced garlic, grated Parmesan cheese, and Italian herbs and spices. Form the mixture into meatballs and bake until golden brown and cooked through. Serve with marinara sauce and whole wheat pasta or zucchini noodles for a delicious and satisfying meal.

7. **Chicken and Rice Casserole**: Combine cooked chicken breast with cooked brown rice, mixed vegetables, and a creamy sauce made from Greek yogurt, chicken broth, and Dijon mustard. Top with shredded cheese and bake until bubbly

and golden brown for a comforting and nutritious casserole option.

8. **Turkey and Sweet Potato Chili**: In a large pot, sauté diced onions, bell peppers, and garlic until softened. Add ground turkey, diced sweet potatoes, canned diced tomatoes, kidney beans, and your favorite chili spices to the pot. Simmer until the sweet potatoes are tender and the flavors meld together for a hearty and flavorful chili.

9. **Chicken and Mushroom Risotto**: Sauté diced chicken breast with sliced mushrooms, onions, and garlic until cooked through. Add Arborio rice and chicken broth to the skillet and simmer until the rice is creamy and tender. Stir in grated Parmesan cheese and chopped fresh herbs for a decadent and comforting risotto.

10. **Turkey and Vegetable Meatloaf**: Mix ground turkey with grated zucchini, carrots, onions, and garlic, along with breadcrumbs, egg, and your favorite herbs and spices. Form the mixture into a loaf and bake until cooked through and golden brown. Serve with mashed sweet potatoes and steamed green beans for a satisfying and nutritious meal.

These comforting chicken and turkey dishes are perfect for beginners on the Galveston Diet who want flavorful and satisfying dinner options that are easy to prepare and packed with nutrition.

CHAPTER EIGHT

Sides and Accompaniments

Incorporating wholesome sides and accompaniments into your meals is essential for creating balanced and satisfying dishes, especially when following the Galveston Diet. In this section, we'll explore a variety of side dishes and accompaniments perfect for beginners on the Galveston Diet, including a beginner's guide to cooking vegetables the Galveston way, easy and healthy grain side dishes, and beginner-friendly bean and legume recipes.

Beginner's Guide to Cooking Vegetables the Galveston Way

Cooking vegetables the Galveston way involves methods that preserve their natural flavors, textures, and nutrients while enhancing their overall appeal. Here's a beginner's guide to cooking vegetables the Galveston way:

1. **Roasting**: Preheat your oven to 400°F (200°C). Toss vegetables like carrots, broccoli, cauliflower, Brussels sprouts, or sweet potatoes with olive oil, salt, and pepper. Spread them out on a baking sheet in a single layer and roast until tender and caramelized, about 20-30 minutes, flipping halfway through.

2. **Steaming**: Fill a pot with a few inches of water and bring it to a simmer over medium heat. Place a steamer basket in the

pot and add vegetables like broccoli, green beans, or asparagus. Cover and steam until vegetables are tender-crisp, about 5-7 minutes.

3. **Sautéing**: Heat a skillet over medium heat and add a bit of olive oil or butter. Add vegetables like bell peppers, zucchini, mushrooms, or spinach to the skillet and cook until tender, stirring occasionally, about 5-7 minutes.

4. **Grilling**: Preheat your grill to medium-high heat. Brush vegetables like eggplant, zucchini, bell peppers, or corn with olive oil and season with salt and pepper. Grill until charred and tender, turning occasionally, about 5-10 minutes.

5. **Stir-Frying**: Heat a wok or large skillet over high heat and add a bit of sesame oil. Add vegetables like snap peas, bok choy, or cabbage to the wok and stir-fry until crisp-tender, about 3-5 minutes.

6. **Raw**: Enjoy vegetables like carrots, cucumber, bell peppers, or cherry tomatoes raw as a crunchy and refreshing addition to salads or as a snack with hummus or Greek yogurt dip.

By using these cooking methods, you can prepare vegetables in a variety of delicious and nutritious ways that complement the Galveston Diet principles.

Easy and Healthy Grain Side Dishes for Beginners

Incorporating whole grains into your meals is a great way to add fiber, vitamins, and minerals to your diet. Here are some easy and healthy grain side dishes for beginners:

1. **Quinoa Pilaf**: Cook quinoa according to package instructions, then fluff with a fork and toss with sautéed vegetables like onions, bell peppers, and spinach. Season with herbs like parsley, thyme, and lemon zest for a flavorful and nutritious side dish.

2. **Brown Rice Salad**: Cook brown rice according to package instructions, then toss with diced vegetables like cucumber, tomatoes, and bell peppers. Dress with a vinaigrette made from olive oil, lemon juice, garlic, and Dijon mustard for a refreshing and colorful side dish.

3. **Farro Risotto**: Cook farro according to package instructions, then simmer in vegetable broth until creamy and tender. Stir in grated Parmesan cheese, sautéed mushrooms, and chopped fresh herbs like parsley and thyme for a hearty and comforting side dish.

4. **Barley and Vegetable Stir-Fry**: Cook barley according to package instructions, then stir-fry with mixed vegetables like snap peas, carrots, and bell peppers in a wok or skillet.

Season with soy sauce, ginger, and garlic for a flavorful and satisfying side dish.

5. **Millet Tabouli**: Cook millet according to package instructions, then toss with chopped parsley, diced tomatoes, cucumber, red onion, and lemon juice. Season with olive oil, salt, and pepper for a refreshing and gluten-free side dish.

6. **Bulgur Salad**: Cook bulgur according to package instructions, then toss with diced vegetables like cherry tomatoes, cucumber, and red onion. Dress with a mixture of olive oil, lemon juice, garlic, and fresh herbs like mint and parsley for a light and summery side dish.

7. **Wild Rice Pilaf**: Cook wild rice according to package instructions, then toss with sautéed mushrooms, dried cranberries, and chopped pecans. Season with a drizzle of maple syrup and a sprinkle of cinnamon for a sweet and savory side dish.

8. **Couscous Tabbouleh**: Cook couscous according to package instructions, then toss with chopped parsley, mint, cucumber, tomatoes, and green onions. Dress with lemon juice, olive oil, garlic, and salt for a refreshing and flavorful side dish.

9. **Sorghum Salad**: Cook sorghum according to package instructions, then toss with diced vegetables like roasted sweet potatoes, red bell peppers, and avocado. Dress with a lime vinaigrette made from lime juice, olive oil, honey, and cumin for a hearty and nutritious side dish.

10. **Rice and Lentil Pilaf**: Cook a mixture of rice and lentils according to package instructions, then toss with sautéed onions, garlic, and carrots. Season with spices like cumin, coriander, and cinnamon for a fragrant and protein-rich side dish.

These easy and healthy grain side dishes are perfect for beginners on the Galveston Diet and can be enjoyed alongside a variety of main courses for a balanced and satisfying meal.

Beginner-Friendly Bean and Legume Recipes

Beans and legumes are nutrient-rich and versatile ingredients that can be incorporated into a variety of dishes. Here are some beginner-friendly bean and legume recipes:

1. **Black Bean and Corn Salad**: Combine canned black beans, cooked corn kernels, diced tomatoes, red onion, and cilantro in a bowl. Dress with lime juice, olive oil, garlic, and cumin for a flavorful and colorful salad option.

2. **Chickpea Salad**: Mix canned chickpeas with diced cucumber, cherry tomatoes, red onion, and parsley in a bowl. Dress

with lemon juice, olive oil, garlic, and oregano for a refreshing and protein-rich salad option.

3. **Lentil Soup**: Cook dried lentils in vegetable broth with diced carrots, celery, onions, and garlic until tender. Season with herbs like thyme, rosemary, and bay leaves for a hearty and comforting soup option.

4. **Black Bean Quesadillas**: Mash canned black beans with salsa, diced onions, and shredded cheese. Spread the bean mixture onto whole grain tortillas, then fold in half and cook in a skillet until crispy and golden for a protein-rich and satisfying meal option.

5. **White Bean Hummus**: Blend canned white beans with garlic, lemon juice, tahini, and olive oil until smooth and creamy. Serve with raw vegetable sticks or whole grain crackers for a delicious and protein-rich snack option.

6. **Red Lentil Curry**: Cook red lentils in coconut milk with diced tomatoes, onions, garlic, ginger, and curry powder until thick and creamy. Serve over cooked brown rice or quinoa for a flavorful and protein-rich curry option.

7. **Chickpea Stir-Fry**: Sauté canned chickpeas with mixed vegetables like bell peppers, broccoli, and snow peas in a wok or skillet. Season with soy sauce, ginger, and garlic for a quick and nutritious stir-fry option.

8. **Black Bean and Quinoa Salad**: Combine cooked quinoa with canned black beans, diced bell peppers, corn kernels, and cilantro in a bowl. Dress with lime juice, olive oil, garlic, and cumin for a protein-rich and flavorful salad option.

9. **Lentil Salad**: Mix cooked lentils with diced cucumber, cherry tomatoes, red onion, and feta cheese in a bowl. Dress with balsamic vinaigrette and fresh herbs like parsley and mint for a refreshing and protein-rich salad option.

10. **Bean and Vegetable Tacos**: Fill whole grain tortillas with cooked beans, sautéed vegetables, shredded lettuce, diced tomatoes, and avocado slices. Serve with salsa and Greek yogurt or sour cream for a delicious and protein-rich taco option.

These beginner-friendly bean and legume recipes are perfect for incorporating nutritious and satisfying ingredients into your meals while following the Galveston Diet principles.

Conclusion

Incorporating wholesome sides and accompaniments into your meals is essential for creating balanced and satisfying dishes, especially when following the Galveston Diet. By using the beginner's guide to cooking vegetables the Galveston way, preparing easy and healthy grain side dishes, and exploring beginner-friendly bean and legume recipes, you can create delicious and nutritious meals that support your health and wellness goals. Whether you're looking for ways to add more vegetables to your diet, incorporate whole grains into your meals, or explore new plant-based protein sources, the options outlined in this section provide a variety of delicious and satisfying choices to enhance your Galveston Diet experience.

CHAPTER NINE

Sweet Treats and Desserts

Indulging in sweet treats and desserts doesn't have to derail your progress on the Galveston Diet. In fact, there are plenty of delicious options that align with the program's principles and satisfy your cravings. In this section, we'll explore a variety of sweet treats and desserts suitable for beginners on the Galveston Diet.

Beginner-Friendly Fruit-Based Desserts

Fruit-based desserts are not only delicious but also packed with vitamins, minerals, and fiber. They're perfect for satisfying your sweet tooth while staying on track with your health goals. Here are some beginner-friendly fruit-based dessert ideas:

1. **Mixed Berry Salad**: Combine fresh strawberries, blueberries, raspberries, and blackberries in a bowl. Drizzle with a bit of honey or maple syrup and sprinkle with chopped mint leaves for a refreshing and naturally sweet dessert.

2. **Fruit Kabobs**: Thread chunks of pineapple, mango, kiwi, and strawberries onto skewers for a fun and colorful dessert option. Serve with a side of Greek yogurt or a drizzle of melted dark chocolate for dipping.

3. **Watermelon Pizza**: Slice a watermelon into rounds and top with Greek yogurt or coconut yogurt. Add sliced

strawberries, kiwi, and blueberries for a colorful and refreshing fruit pizza that's as delicious as it is eye-catching.

4. **Frozen Banana Pops**: Insert popsicle sticks into peeled bananas and freeze until firm. Dip the frozen bananas in melted dark chocolate and sprinkle with chopped nuts or shredded coconut for a satisfying and naturally sweet treat.

5. **Stuffed Dates**: Remove the pits from Medjool dates and fill them with almond butter or cashew butter. Sprinkle with a pinch of sea salt or cinnamon for a sweet and indulgent snack that's perfect for satisfying cravings.

6. **Grilled Fruit**: Grill slices of pineapple, peaches, or plums until caramelized and tender. Serve with a dollop of Greek yogurt or a scoop of vanilla ice cream for a simple yet decadent dessert option.

7. **Baked Apples**: Core apples and fill the center with a mixture of oats, nuts, cinnamon, and a drizzle of honey or maple syrup. Bake until the apples are tender and the filling is golden brown for a warm and comforting dessert.

8. **Fruit Salsa with Cinnamon Chips**: Dice mangoes, strawberries, and kiwi and toss them with a squeeze of lime juice and a sprinkle of cinnamon. Serve with homemade cinnamon chips made from whole grain tortillas for a flavorful and crunchy dessert option.

9. **Berry Parfait**: Layer Greek yogurt with mixed berries and granola in parfait glasses for a simple yet satisfying dessert that's perfect for breakfast or anytime you need a sweet treat.

10.   **Frozen Fruit Bars**: Puree mixed fruits like strawberries, raspberries, and peaches with a bit of honey or agave syrup. Pour the mixture into popsicle molds and freeze until firm for a refreshing and naturally sweet frozen treat.

These beginner-friendly fruit-based desserts are not only delicious but also nutritious, making them a perfect choice for satisfying your sweet cravings while following the Galveston Diet.

Simple and Delicious Galveston Diet Dessert Recipes for Beginners

Creating homemade desserts allows you to control the ingredients and make healthier choices that align with the Galveston Diet principles. Here are some simple and delicious dessert recipes that are perfect for beginners:

1. **Chocolate Avocado Pudding**: Blend ripe avocados with cocoa powder, almond milk, honey or maple syrup, and a splash of vanilla extract until smooth and creamy. Chill in the refrigerator for a few hours until set for a rich and indulgent chocolate pudding.

2. **Coconut Chia Seed Pudding**: Mix coconut milk with chia seeds, honey or agave syrup, and a splash of vanilla extract in a jar. Refrigerate overnight until thickened, then top with fresh berries or toasted coconut for a creamy and satisfying pudding option.

3. **Banana Chocolate Chip Muffins**: Mash ripe bananas and mix them with whole wheat flour, almond milk, honey or maple syrup, cinnamon, and dark chocolate chips. Spoon the batter into muffin cups and bake until golden brown for a wholesome and delicious treat.

4. **Berry Crisp**: Toss mixed berries with a bit of honey or maple syrup and place them in a baking dish. Top with a mixture of rolled oats, almond flour, coconut oil, cinnamon, and a pinch of salt, then bake until bubbly and golden brown for a comforting and nutritious dessert.

5. **Peanut Butter Energy Balls**: Mix rolled oats with peanut butter, honey or agave syrup, chia seeds, and a pinch of salt. Roll the mixture into balls and refrigerate until firm for a convenient and energy-boosting snack or dessert option.

6. **Almond Flour Banana Bread**: Combine almond flour with mashed bananas, eggs, honey or maple syrup, cinnamon, and baking powder. Pour the batter into a loaf pan and bake until golden brown and cooked through for a moist and flavorful banana bread.

7. **Greek Yogurt Bark**: Spread Greek yogurt onto a baking sheet lined with parchment paper, then top with sliced strawberries, blueberries, and a sprinkle of granola. Freeze until firm, then break into pieces for a refreshing and customizable dessert option.

8. **Chocolate Covered Strawberries**: Dip fresh strawberries in melted dark chocolate and let them set on a parchment-lined baking sheet. Enjoy these elegant and indulgent treats as a satisfying dessert or snack option.

9. **Lemon Poppy Seed Muffins**: Combine whole wheat flour with almond milk, lemon zest, lemon juice, honey or agave syrup, poppy seeds, and baking powder. Spoon the batter into muffin cups and bake until lightly golden and cooked through for a bright and citrusy treat.

10. **Apple Cinnamon Oat Bars**: Mix rolled oats with diced apples, cinnamon, honey or maple syrup, and a pinch of salt. Press the mixture into a baking dish and bake until golden brown and crisp for a wholesome and satisfying dessert option.

These simple and delicious Galveston Diet dessert recipes are perfect for beginners and allow you to enjoy sweet treats without compromising your health goals.

Indulgent Yet Healthy Desserts for Beginner Galveston Dieters

Indulging in dessert doesn't have to mean sacrificing your health goals. With the right ingredients and recipes, you can enjoy indulgent yet healthy desserts that satisfy your cravings without the guilt. Here are some ideas for indulgent yet healthy desserts suitable for beginner Galveston dieters:

1. **Avocado Chocolate Mousse**: Blend ripe avocados with cocoa powder, honey or maple syrup, vanilla extract, and a pinch of salt until smooth and creamy. Chill in the refrigerator until set for a rich and decadent chocolate mousse that's packed with healthy fats and antioxidants.

2. **Chia Seed Chocolate Pudding**: Mix chia seeds with almond milk, cocoa powder, honey or agave syrup, and a splash of vanilla extract in a jar. Refrigerate overnight until thickened, then top with sliced bananas or berries for a creamy and nutritious dessert option.

3. **Frozen Yogurt Bark**: Spread Greek yogurt onto a baking sheet lined with parchment paper, then top with sliced fruit, nuts, and a drizzle of honey or maple syrup. Freeze until firm, then break into pieces for a refreshing and protein-rich dessert option.

4. **Coconut Date Balls**: Blend dates with shredded coconut, almond flour, vanilla extract, and a pinch of salt until smooth. Roll the mixture into balls and coat them in shredded coconut or chopped nuts for a sweet and satisfying snack or dessert option.

5. **Chocolate Covered Almonds**: Dip roasted almonds in melted dark chocolate and let them set on a parchment-lined baking sheet. Enjoy these crunchy and chocolatey treats as a nutritious snack or dessert option.

6. **Baked Pears with Honey and Cinnamon**: Core pears and drizzle them with honey or maple syrup, cinnamon, and a sprinkle of chopped nuts. Bake until tender and caramelized for a warm and comforting dessert option that's naturally sweet and satisfying.

7. **Banana Nice Cream**: Blend frozen bananas with a splash of almond milk, vanilla extract, and a pinch of cinnamon until smooth and creamy. Serve immediately for a dairy-free and naturally sweet alternative to traditional ice cream.

8. **Almond Butter Cups**: Mix almond butter with cocoa powder, honey or agave syrup, and a pinch of salt until smooth. Spoon the mixture into mini muffin cups lined with parchment paper and freeze until set for a satisfying and protein-rich dessert option.

9. **Baked Apples with Cinnamon and Walnuts**: Core apples and fill them with a mixture of chopped walnuts, cinnamon, honey or maple syrup, and a splash of lemon juice. Bake until tender and fragrant for a warm and comforting dessert option that's perfect for chilly evenings.

10. **Dark Chocolate-Dipped Strawberries**: Dip fresh strawberries in melted dark chocolate and let them set on a parchment-lined baking sheet. Enjoy these elegant and indulgent treats as a satisfying dessert or snack option.

These indulgent yet healthy dessert options are perfect for beginner Galveston dieters who want to satisfy their sweet cravings without compromising their health goals. Enjoy these treats in moderation as part of a balanced diet and lifestyle.

CHAPTER TEN

Lifestyle Tips and Tricks for Success

Navigating a healthy lifestyle goes beyond just dietary choices; it involves incorporating various habits and practices that support overall well-being. In this section, we'll delve into lifestyle tips and tricks for success on the Galveston Diet, covering topics such as incorporating exercise into your journey, stress management and mindful eating techniques, and building healthy habits for long-term success.

Incorporating Exercise into Your Galveston Diet Journey

Exercise is a crucial component of a healthy lifestyle and complements the dietary principles of the Galveston Diet. Here are some tips for incorporating exercise into your Galveston Diet journey:

1. **Find Activities You Enjoy**: Explore different types of physical activity, such as walking, cycling, swimming, yoga, or dancing, and choose activities that you genuinely enjoy. This will make it easier to stay consistent and motivated.

2. **Start Slowly and Progress Gradually**: If you're new to exercise or have been inactive for a while, start with low-impact activities and gradually increase the intensity and duration as your fitness level improves. Listen to your body

and avoid pushing yourself too hard, especially in the beginning.

3. **Schedule Regular Workouts**: Treat exercise like any other important appointment and schedule it into your daily or weekly routine. Consistency is key, so aim for at least 30 minutes of moderate-intensity exercise most days of the week.

4. **Combine Cardiovascular and Strength Training**: Include a mix of cardiovascular exercises, such as brisk walking, jogging, or cycling, with strength training exercises, such as bodyweight exercises, weightlifting, or resistance band workouts, to improve overall fitness and health.

5. **Set Realistic Goals**: Set specific, measurable, achievable, relevant, and time-bound (SMART) goals for your exercise routine. Whether it's completing a certain number of workouts per week, increasing your strength or endurance, or participating in a fitness event, having clear goals can help keep you motivated and focused.

6. **Mix It Up**: Keep your workouts interesting and challenging by trying new activities, varying the intensity or duration of your workouts, or incorporating different types of exercises into your routine. This prevents boredom and plateaus while providing a well-rounded fitness experience.

7. **Stay Active Throughout the Day**: Look for opportunities to be active throughout the day, such as taking the stairs instead of the elevator, parking farther away from your destination, or doing household chores or gardening. Every little bit of movement adds up and contributes to your overall physical activity level.

8. **Listen to Your Body**: Pay attention to how your body responds to exercise and adjust your routine accordingly. If you experience pain, discomfort, or fatigue, take a break or modify your workout to prevent injury and promote recovery.

9. **Stay Hydrated and Fuel Your Body**: Drink plenty of water before, during, and after exercise to stay hydrated, and fuel your body with nutritious foods that provide the energy and nutrients needed for optimal performance and recovery.

10. **Celebrate Your Progress**: Celebrate your achievements and milestones along your fitness journey, whether it's reaching a new personal best, completing a challenging workout, or consistently sticking to your exercise routine. Acknowledging your progress can boost motivation and confidence.

Incorporating regular exercise into your Galveston Diet journey not only supports weight management and physical health but also enhances mood, energy levels, and overall well-being.

Stress Management and Mindful Eating Techniques for Beginners

Managing stress and practicing mindful eating are essential components of a balanced lifestyle and can positively impact your relationship with food and overall health. Here are some tips for incorporating stress management and mindful eating techniques into your routine as a beginner:

1. **Practice Deep Breathing**: Incorporate deep breathing exercises into your daily routine to reduce stress and promote relaxation. Take slow, deep breaths, focusing on filling your lungs with air and exhaling slowly. This can help calm the nervous system and alleviate feelings of tension or anxiety.

2. **Engage in Stress-Relieving Activities**: Find activities that help you unwind and de-stress, such as meditation, yoga, tai chi, mindfulness practices, or spending time in nature. Experiment with different techniques to discover what works best for you and make them a regular part of your routine.

3. **Prioritize Sleep**: Aim for 7-9 hours of quality sleep per night to support overall health and well-being. Create a relaxing bedtime routine, avoid screens and stimulating activities before bed, and create a comfortable sleep environment to promote restful sleep.

4. **Practice Mindful Eating**: Pay attention to your eating habits and cultivate mindfulness around food. Slow down and savor each bite, paying attention to the taste, texture, and aroma of your food. Notice hunger and fullness cues and eat until you feel satisfied, rather than overly full.

5. **Eat Without Distractions**: Minimize distractions while eating, such as watching TV, scrolling on your phone, or working at your desk. Instead, create a calm and focused eating environment, free from distractions, to fully enjoy and appreciate your meals.

6. **Listen to Your Body**: Tune into your body's hunger and fullness signals and honor its cues for nourishment. Eat when you're hungry and stop when you're satisfied, rather than eating out of boredom, stress, or habit.

7. **Choose Nutrient-Dense Foods**: Focus on including a variety of nutrient-dense foods in your diet, such as fruits, vegetables, whole grains, lean proteins, and healthy fats. These foods provide essential nutrients and support overall health and well-being.

8. **Practice Gratitude**: Cultivate an attitude of gratitude and appreciation for the food you eat and the nourishment it provides. Take a moment before meals to express gratitude for the flavors, textures, and nourishment of your food.

9. **Be Kind to Yourself**: Practice self-compassion and kindness towards yourself, especially when it comes to your relationship with food and body image. Let go of perfectionism and embrace a mindset of progress over perfection.

10.   **Seek Support if Needed**: If you're struggling with stress management or mindful eating, don't hesitate to seek support from a qualified healthcare professional, therapist, or registered dietitian. They can provide guidance, tools, and resources to help you develop healthy coping strategies and improve your relationship with food.

By incorporating stress management techniques and mindful eating practices into your daily life, you can cultivate a healthier relationship with food, reduce stress, and promote overall well-being on your Galveston Diet journey.

Building Healthy Habits for Long-Term Success

Building healthy habits is essential for long-term success on the Galveston Diet and beyond. Here are some tips for establishing and maintaining healthy habits as a beginner:

1. **Start Small**: Focus on making small, sustainable changes to your lifestyle rather than trying to overhaul everything at once. Choose one or two habits to work on at a time, such as drinking more water, adding more vegetables to your meals, or going for a daily walk.

2. **Set Clear Goals**: Define specific and achievable goals for yourself, whether it's related to nutrition, exercise, stress management, or other aspects of your health and well-being. Break larger goals into smaller, actionable steps and track your progress along the way.

3. **Create a Routine**: Establish a consistent daily routine that includes healthy habits such as regular mealtimes, dedicated time for exercise or physical activity, adequate sleep, and stress management practices. Consistency is key to forming lasting habits.

4. **Use Visual Reminders**: Place visual reminders of your goals and intentions in prominent places where you'll see them regularly, such as on your fridge, bathroom mirror, or desktop. This can help reinforce your commitment to making healthy choices.

5. **Find an Accountability Partner**: Partner with a friend, family member, or coworker who shares similar health goals and support each other in staying accountable. Check in regularly to share progress, celebrate successes, and troubleshoot challenges together.

6. **Practice Self-Reflection**: Take time to reflect on your habits, behaviors, and progress regularly. Identify what's working well and what areas may need improvement, and make adjustments as needed to stay on track with your goals.

7. **Stay Flexible**: Be willing to adapt and adjust your habits as needed based on changes in your schedule, preferences, or circumstances. Life can be unpredictable, so having flexibility and resilience is essential for maintaining healthy habits over the long term.

8. **Celebrate Milestones**: Celebrate your achievements and milestones along the way, no matter how small. Whether it's reaching a certain weight loss goal, sticking to your exercise routine for a month, or mastering a new healthy recipe, take time to acknowledge and celebrate your progress.

9. **Practice Patience and Persistence**: Building healthy habits takes time, patience, and persistence. Be kind to yourself and recognize that change doesn't happen overnight. Focus on progress rather than perfection and keep moving forward, even when faced with setbacks or challenges.

10. **Stay Motivated**: Find sources of inspiration and motivation to keep you focused on your goals. This could include reading success stories, following inspiring individuals on social media, joining online communities or support groups, or seeking out new challenges and experiences to keep things fresh and exciting.

By building healthy habits and incorporating them into your daily routine, you can create a solid foundation for long-term success on the Galveston Diet and enjoy improved health and well-being for years to come.

CHAPTER 11

A 31 DAY MEAL PLAN

Week 1:

Day 1:

- Breakfast: Scrambled eggs with spinach and mushrooms.

- Lunch: Grilled chicken salad with mixed greens, cherry tomatoes, and avocado.

- Dinner: Baked salmon with roasted asparagus and quinoa.

Day 2:

- Breakfast: Greek yogurt with sliced almonds and berries.

- Lunch: Turkey and avocado wrap with whole wheat tortilla.

- Dinner: Lemon herb grilled chicken breast with roasted Brussels sprouts and sweet potatoes.

Day 3:

- Breakfast: Oatmeal topped with sliced bananas and a drizzle of honey.

- Lunch: Mediterranean quinoa salad with cucumber, tomatoes, red onion, and feta cheese.

- Dinner: Grilled shrimp skewers with quinoa tabbouleh.

Day 4:

- Breakfast: Whole grain toast with mashed avocado and poached eggs.

- Lunch: Tuna salad with mixed greens, cherry tomatoes, and olives.

- Dinner: Baked cod with lemon and herbs, served with steamed broccoli.

Day 5:

- Breakfast: Smoothie made with spinach, banana, Greek yogurt, and almond milk.

- Lunch: Hummus and vegetable wrap with whole wheat tortilla.

- Dinner: Turkey meatballs with marinara sauce, served over zucchini noodles.

Day 6:

- Breakfast: Greek yogurt parfait with granola and mixed berries.

- Lunch: Greek salad with grilled chicken breast and balsamic vinaigrette.

- Dinner: Baked tilapia with Mediterranean roasted vegetables.

Day 7:

- Breakfast: Scrambled eggs with diced bell peppers and onions.

- Lunch: Caprese salad with tomato, mozzarella, basil, and balsamic glaze.

- Dinner: Turkey chili with black beans and corn.

Week 2:

Day 8:

- Breakfast: Whole grain pancakes with sliced peaches and Greek yogurt.

- Lunch: Greek yogurt tzatziki dip with whole grain pita chips and carrot sticks.

- Dinner: Grilled lemon garlic shrimp with quinoa and roasted asparagus.

Day 9:

- Breakfast: Omelette with spinach, mushrooms, and feta cheese.

- Lunch: Mediterranean chickpea salad with cucumber, red onion, and parsley.

- Dinner: Baked chicken thighs with Mediterranean couscous.

Day 10:

- Breakfast: Greek yogurt with honey and chopped walnuts.

- Lunch: Mediterranean quinoa tabbouleh salad with diced vegetables and herbs.

- Dinner: Grilled lamb chops with roasted sweet potatoes and green beans.

Day 11:

- Breakfast: Whole grain toast with almond butter and sliced bananas.

- Lunch: Greek salad with cucumber, tomato, olives, and feta cheese.

- Dinner: Lemon herb grilled swordfish with quinoa and steamed broccoli.

Day 12:

- Breakfast: Smoothie bowl topped with granola, sliced strawberries, and honey.

- Lunch: Turkey and avocado wrap with whole wheat tortilla.

- Dinner: Baked cod with tomatoes, olives, and capers, served with roasted potatoes.

Day 13:

- Breakfast: Greek yogurt parfait with granola and mixed berries.

- Lunch: Hummus and vegetable wrap with whole wheat tortilla.

- Dinner: Baked chicken breast with Mediterranean quinoa salad.

Day 14:

- Breakfast: Scrambled eggs with diced bell peppers and onions.

- Lunch: Caprese salad with tomato, mozzarella, basil, and balsamic glaze.

- Dinner: Turkey chili with black beans and corn.

Week 3:

Day 15:

- Breakfast: Whole grain pancakes with sliced peaches and Greek yogurt.

- Lunch: Greek yogurt tzatziki dip with whole grain pita chips and carrot sticks.

- Dinner: Grilled lemon garlic shrimp with quinoa and roasted asparagus.

Day 16:

- Breakfast: Omelette with spinach, mushrooms, and feta cheese.

- Lunch: Mediterranean chickpea salad with cucumber, red onion, and parsley.

- Dinner: Baked chicken thighs with Mediterranean couscous.

Day 17:

- Breakfast: Greek yogurt with honey and chopped walnuts.

- Lunch: Mediterranean quinoa tabbouleh salad with diced vegetables and herbs.

- Dinner: Grilled lamb chops with roasted sweet potatoes and green beans.

Day 18:

- Breakfast: Whole grain toast with almond butter and sliced bananas.

- Lunch: Greek salad with cucumber, tomato, olives, and feta cheese.

- Dinner: Lemon herb grilled swordfish with quinoa and steamed broccoli.

Day 19:

- Breakfast: Smoothie bowl topped with granola, sliced strawberries, and honey.

- Lunch: Turkey and avocado wrap with whole wheat tortilla.

- Dinner: Baked cod with tomatoes, olives, and capers, served with roasted potatoes.

Day 20:

- Breakfast: Greek yogurt parfait with granola and mixed berries.

- Lunch: Hummus and vegetable wrap with whole wheat tortilla.

- Dinner: Baked chicken breast with Mediterranean quinoa salad.

Day 21:

- Breakfast: Scrambled eggs with diced bell peppers and onions.

- Lunch: Caprese salad with tomato, mozzarella, basil, and balsamic glaze.

- Dinner: Turkey chili with black beans and corn.

Week 4:

Day 22:

- Breakfast: Whole grain pancakes with sliced peaches and Greek yogurt.

- Lunch: Greek yogurt tzatziki dip with whole grain pita chips and carrot sticks.

- Dinner: Grilled lemon garlic shrimp with quinoa and roasted asparagus.

Day 23:

- Breakfast: Omelette with spinach, mushrooms, and feta cheese.

- Lunch: Mediterranean chickpea salad with cucumber, red onion, and parsley.

- Dinner: Baked chicken thighs with Mediterranean couscous.

Day 24:

- Breakfast: Greek yogurt with honey and chopped walnuts.

- Lunch: Mediterranean quinoa tabbouleh salad with diced vegetables and herbs.

- Dinner: Grilled lamb chops with roasted sweet potatoes and green beans.

Day 25:

- Breakfast: Whole grain toast with almond butter and sliced bananas.

- Lunch: Greek salad with cucumber, tomato, olives, and feta cheese.

- Dinner: Lemon herb grilled swordfish with quinoa and steamed broccoli.

Day 26:

- Breakfast: Smoothie bowl topped with granola, sliced strawberries, and honey.
- Lunch: Turkey and avocado wrap with whole wheat tortilla.
- Dinner: Baked cod with tomatoes, olives, and capers, served with roasted potatoes.

Day 27:

- Breakfast: Greek yogurt parfait with granola and mixed berries.
- Lunch: Hummus and vegetable wrap with whole wheat tortilla.
- Dinner: Baked chicken breast with Mediterranean quinoa salad.

Day 28:

- Breakfast: Scrambled eggs with diced bell peppers and onions.
- Lunch: Caprese salad with tomato, mozzarella, basil, and balsamic glaze.
- Dinner: Turkey chili with black beans and corn.

Day 29:

- Breakfast: Whole grain pancakes with sliced peaches and Greek yogurt.

- Lunch: Greek yogurt tzatziki dip with whole grain pita chips and carrot sticks.

- Dinner: Grilled lemon garlic shrimp with quinoa and roasted asparagus.

Day 30:

- Breakfast: Omelette with spinach, mushrooms, and feta cheese.

- Lunch: Mediterranean chickpea salad with cucumber, red onion, and parsley.

- Dinner: Baked chicken thighs with Mediterranean couscous.

Day 31:

- Breakfast: Greek yogurt with honey and chopped walnuts.

- Lunch: Mediterranean quinoa tabbouleh salad with diced vegetables and herbs.

- Dinner: Grilled lamb chops with roasted sweet potatoes and green beans.

BONUS: SOME ESSENTIAL RECIPES FOR HEALTH AND WELLNESS

Cucumbers Diet

Definition: The cucumbers diet emphasizes the consumption of cucumbers as a primary vegetable in meals or snacks. Cucumbers are low in calories, refreshing, and hydrating, making them an excellent choice for those looking to increase vegetable intake, support hydration, and promote weight loss or management.

Ingredients:

- **Cucumbers:** The star ingredient, low in calories and high in water content, serves as the foundation of this diet.

- **Dressing or Dip:** Pair cucumbers with healthy dressings or dips such as hummus, Greek yogurt-based dips, or vinaigrettes for added flavor and creaminess.

- **Proteins:** Combine cucumbers with protein sources like grilled chicken, tofu, or chickpeas to create balanced and satisfying meals.

- **Whole Grains:** Serve cucumbers alongside whole grains like quinoa, brown rice, or farro for added fiber and sustained energy.

- **Herbs and Spices:** Flavor cucumbers with herbs, spices, or seasonings like mint, dill, or lemon zest to enhance taste and aroma.

Instructions:

1. **Simple Snack:** Enjoy sliced cucumbers on their own as a refreshing and hydrating snack option.

2. **Salads:** Incorporate cucumbers into salads alongside other vegetables, greens, proteins, and grains for a nutritious and filling meal.

3. **Cucumber Cups:** Use cucumber slices or hollowed-out cucumber halves as cups to hold fillings like tuna salad, chicken salad, or hummus for a fun and creative appetizer or snack.

4. **Pickles:** Make homemade pickles by soaking cucumber slices in a mixture of vinegar, water, salt, and spices for a tangy and crunchy snack.

5. **Cucumber Water:** Infuse water with cucumber slices and fresh herbs like mint or basil for a refreshing and hydrating beverage option.

Egg Diet

Definition: The egg diet involves incorporating eggs as a primary source of protein in meals. Eggs are nutrient-dense, rich in high-quality protein, vitamins, minerals, and healthy fats. This diet is often used for weight loss, muscle building, or as part of a balanced eating plan.

Ingredients:

- **Eggs:** The main ingredient, providing high-quality protein, essential vitamins (such as vitamin B12 and vitamin D), and minerals (such as iron and selenium).

- **Vegetables:** Pair eggs with a variety of vegetables like spinach, bell peppers, tomatoes, or mushrooms for added fiber, vitamins, and minerals.

- **Whole Grains:** Serve eggs alongside whole grains such as whole wheat toast, quinoa, or oatmeal for sustained energy and additional fiber.

- **Healthy Fats:** Incorporate sources of healthy fats like avocado, olive oil, nuts, or seeds to enhance satiety and nutrient absorption.

- **Herbs and Spices:** Flavor egg dishes with herbs, spices, and seasonings like black pepper, paprika, or fresh herbs to add depth and complexity to the flavors.

Instructions:

1. **Basic Preparation:** Enjoy eggs cooked in various ways, such as boiled, poached, scrambled, fried (using minimal oil), or baked, depending on personal preference.

2. **Omelets:** Make omelets by whisking eggs with vegetables, cheese, and herbs, then cooking them in a skillet until set. Customize omelets with your favorite fillings for a nutritious and satisfying meal.

3. **Frittatas:** Bake eggs with vegetables and cheese in a frittata for a simple and versatile dish that can be enjoyed for breakfast, lunch, or dinner.

4. **Egg Salad:** Prepare egg salad by mixing chopped hard-boiled eggs with Greek yogurt, mustard, celery, and spices. Serve on whole grain bread or lettuce wraps for a protein-rich meal.

5. **Meal Prep:** Boil a batch of eggs in advance and store them in the fridge for easy meal prep throughout the week. Hard-boiled eggs make a convenient and portable snack or addition to salads and sandwiches.

Fish Diet

Definition: The fish diet involves incorporating various types of fish into meals to reap the health benefits associated with consuming seafood. Fish is rich in high-quality protein, omega-3 fatty acids, vitamins, and minerals, making it a valuable component of a healthy eating plan.

Ingredients:

- **Fish:** Choose a variety of fish species such as salmon, tuna, trout, mackerel, sardines, or cod to enjoy a diverse range of flavors and nutrients.

- **Vegetables:** Pair fish with a variety of vegetables like leafy greens, broccoli, asparagus, or zucchini for added fiber, vitamins, and minerals.

- **Whole Grains:** Serve fish alongside whole grains like brown rice, quinoa, or barley for sustained energy and additional fiber.

- **Healthy Fats:** Fish itself is a source of healthy fats, particularly omega-3 fatty acids, which are beneficial for heart health. Supplement with additional sources of healthy fats like avocado, olive oil, nuts, or seeds as desired.

- **Herbs and Spices:** Flavor fish dishes with herbs, spices, and seasonings like garlic, lemon, dill, or thyme to enhance taste and aroma.

Instructions:

1. **Grilled Fish:** Grill fish fillets or whole fish with a drizzle of olive oil and a sprinkle of herbs and spices for a simple and flavorful dish.

2. **Baked Fish:** Bake fish fillets with lemon slices, garlic, and herbs for a light and healthy meal that's easy to prepare.

3. **Fish Tacos:** Prepare fish tacos by grilling or baking fish, then serving it in corn or whole wheat tortillas with cabbage slaw, avocado, salsa, and a squeeze of lime for a delicious and nutritious meal.

4. **Fish Curry:** Make fish curry by simmering fish with coconut milk, tomatoes, onions, and spices for a flavorful and comforting dish that pairs well with rice or naan.

5. **Canned Fish:** Incorporate canned fish like tuna or salmon into salads, sandwiches, or pasta dishes for a convenient and budget-friendly protein option that's rich in omega-3 fatty acids.

Flaxseeds Diet

Definition: The flaxseeds diet involves incorporating flaxseeds as a nutritional powerhouse into meals to boost fiber, protein, omega-3 fatty acids, and various micronutrients. Flaxseeds are versatile and can be easily added to a wide range of dishes, making them a convenient addition to any diet.

Ingredients:

- **Flaxseeds:** The star ingredient, rich in fiber, protein, omega-3 fatty acids, and antioxidants.

- **Liquid:** Mix ground flaxseeds with liquids such as water, milk (dairy or plant-based), yogurt, or fruit juice to create a flaxseed gel or add them directly into smoothies, oatmeal, or yogurt for added nutrition.

- **Fruits:** Pair flaxseeds with fruits like berries, bananas, or apples for added flavor, sweetness, and additional nutrients.

- **Nuts and Seeds:** Combine flaxseeds with nuts or seeds such as almonds, walnuts, or pumpkin seeds for added texture and nutritional variety.

- **Sweeteners (Optional):** Add natural sweeteners like honey, maple syrup, or agave nectar if desired, but keep in mind the added sugar content.

Instructions:

1. **Flaxseed Gel:** Mix ground flaxseeds with water to create a flaxseed gel, which can be used as an egg substitute in baking recipes or as a thickening agent in sauces and dressings.

2. **Smoothies:** Blend ground flaxseeds into smoothies along with fruits, leafy greens, protein powder, and your choice of liquid for a nutritious and filling beverage rich in omega-3 fatty acids and fiber.

3. **Oatmeal:** Stir ground flaxseeds into cooked oatmeal along with fruits, nuts, and spices for a hearty and nutritious breakfast option.

4. **Baking:** Incorporate ground flaxseeds into baked goods like muffins, bread, or energy bars for added nutrition and texture. Flaxseeds can be used as an egg substitute in vegan baking recipes.

5. **Yogurt Topping:** Sprinkle ground flaxseeds over Greek yogurt along with fruits, nuts, and a drizzle of honey or maple syrup for a nutritious and satisfying snack or breakfast option.

Greek Yogurt Diet

Definition: The Greek yogurt diet involves incorporating Greek yogurt as a central component of meals or snacks due to its high protein content, probiotics, and versatility. Greek yogurt is a strained yogurt that has a thicker consistency and higher protein content compared to regular yogurt, making it a popular choice for those seeking to increase protein intake and support gut health.

Ingredients:

- **Greek Yogurt:** The main ingredient, rich in protein, probiotics, calcium, and other essential nutrients.

- **Fruits:** Pair Greek yogurt with fruits like berries, peaches, or mangoes for added flavor, natural sweetness, and additional vitamins and minerals.

- **Nuts and Seeds:** Combine Greek yogurt with nuts or seeds such as almonds, walnuts, or chia seeds for added texture, healthy fats, and nutritional variety.

- **Honey or Maple Syrup (Optional):** Add natural sweeteners like honey or maple syrup to Greek yogurt if desired, but keep in mind the added sugar content.

- **Whole Grains:** Serve Greek yogurt alongside whole grains like granola, oats, or whole grain cereal for added fiber and sustained energy.

Instructions:

1. **Simple Snack:** Enjoy Greek yogurt on its own as a quick and convenient snack option.

2. **Parfait:** Layer Greek yogurt with your favorite fruits, nuts, seeds, and a drizzle of honey or maple syrup to create a delicious and nutritious parfait.

3. **Smoothies:** Blend Greek yogurt into smoothies along with fruits, leafy greens, protein powder, and your choice of liquid for a protein-rich beverage that's creamy and satisfying.

4. **Salad Dressing:** Use Greek yogurt as a base for salad dressings by mixing it with lemon juice, herbs, spices, and a touch of olive oil for a creamy and tangy dressing option.

5. **Dips:** Combine Greek yogurt with herbs, spices, and seasonings to create savory dips for vegetables, crackers, or pita bread. Greek yogurt-based dips are a healthier alternative to sour cream-based dips and are rich in protein and probiotics.

Green Beans Diet

Definition: The green beans diet involves incorporating green beans as a primary vegetable in meals to boost nutrition and add variety to the diet. Green beans are low in calories, rich in fiber, vitamins (such as vitamin C, vitamin K, and folate), and minerals (such as manganese and potassium), making them a valuable addition to any healthy eating plan.

Ingredients:

- **Green Beans:** The star ingredient, low in calories and high in fiber, vitamins, and minerals, serves as the foundation of this diet.

- **Proteins:** Pair green beans with proteins like grilled chicken, tofu, fish, or lean beef to create balanced and satisfying meals.

- **Whole Grains:** Serve green beans alongside whole grains like quinoa, brown rice, or whole wheat pasta for added fiber and sustained energy.

- **Healthy Fats:** Incorporate sources of healthy fats such as olive oil, avocado, nuts, or seeds to enhance nutrient absorption and satiety.

- **Herbs and Spices:** Flavor green beans with herbs, spices, and seasonings like garlic, lemon, dill, or thyme to enhance taste and aroma.

Instructions:

1. **Steamed Green Beans:** Steam green beans until tender-crisp and season with a sprinkle of salt, pepper, and a drizzle of olive oil for a simple and nutritious side dish.

2. **Green Bean Salad:** Blanch green beans in boiling water, then toss with cherry tomatoes, red onion, feta cheese, and a balsamic vinaigrette for a refreshing and colorful salad.

3. **Stir-Fry:** Stir-fry green beans with garlic, ginger, soy sauce, and your choice of protein for a quick and flavorful Asian-inspired dish.

4. **Roasted Green Beans:** Roast green beans in the oven with olive oil, garlic, and Parmesan cheese for a crispy and savory side dish that pairs well with grilled meats or fish.

5. **Green Bean Casserole:** Prepare a classic green bean casserole with green beans, cream of mushroom soup, and crispy fried onions for a comforting and nostalgic dish that's perfect for holidays or special occasions.

Kale Diet

Definition: The kale diet emphasizes the consumption of kale as a nutrient-rich leafy green vegetable in meals or snacks. Kale is packed with vitamins, minerals, fiber, and antioxidants, making it one of the healthiest foods you can eat.

Ingredients:

- **Kale:** The star ingredient, rich in vitamins (such as vitamin A, vitamin K, and vitamin C), minerals (such as calcium and potassium), fiber, and antioxidants.

- **Fruits:** Pair kale with fruits like berries, apples, or oranges for added flavor, sweetness, and additional nutrients.

- **Nuts and Seeds:** Combine kale with nuts or seeds such as almonds, walnuts, or sunflower seeds for added texture, healthy fats, and nutritional variety.

- **Whole Grains:** Serve kale alongside whole grains like quinoa, farro, or barley for added fiber and sustained energy.

- **Proteins:** Pair kale with proteins like grilled chicken, salmon, tofu, or chickpeas to create balanced and satisfying meals.

Instructions:

1. **Kale Salad:** Massage kale with lemon juice and olive oil to soften the leaves, then toss with your favorite toppings such as avocado, nuts, seeds, and a flavorful dressing for a nutritious and satisfying salad.

2. **Kale Smoothie:** Blend kale into smoothies along with fruits, Greek yogurt, nut milk, and a scoop of protein powder for a green smoothie that's packed with vitamins, minerals, and fiber.

3. **Kale Chips:** Toss kale leaves with olive oil, salt, and your choice of seasonings, then bake in the oven until crispy for a healthy and crunchy snack alternative to potato chips.

4. **Kale Soup:** Simmer kale with vegetables, beans, and broth to create a hearty and nutritious soup that's perfect for cold weather or when you're feeling under the weather.

5. **Stir-Fry:** Stir-fry kale with garlic, ginger, soy sauce, and your choice of protein for a quick and flavorful Asian-inspired dish that's perfect for busy weeknights.

Kiwi Diet

Definition: The kiwi diet involves incorporating kiwi fruit as a primary source of vitamins, minerals, and antioxidants into meals or snacks. Kiwi is renowned for its high vitamin C content, as well as its fiber, potassium, and vitamin K, making it a nutritious addition to any diet.

Ingredients:

- **Kiwi:** The star ingredient, rich in vitamin C, fiber, potassium, and antioxidants, serves as the foundation of this diet.

- **Other Fruits:** Pair kiwi with other fruits such as berries, oranges, or pineapple for added flavor, sweetness, and variety.

- **Greek Yogurt:** Combine kiwi with Greek yogurt for a creamy and nutritious breakfast or snack option that's rich in protein and probiotics.

- **Nuts and Seeds:** Sprinkle chopped kiwi over nuts or seeds like almonds, walnuts, or chia seeds for added texture, healthy fats, and nutritional variety.

- **Whole Grains:** Serve kiwi alongside whole grains like oatmeal, quinoa, or whole grain toast for added fiber and sustained energy.

Instructions:

1. **Kiwi Salad:** Combine sliced kiwi with mixed greens, avocado, nuts, seeds, and a balsamic vinaigrette for a refreshing and nutrient-rich salad.

2. **Kiwi Smoothie:** Blend kiwi into smoothies along with other fruits, leafy greens, Greek yogurt, nut milk, and a scoop of protein powder for a green smoothie that's packed with vitamins, minerals, and protein.

3. **Kiwi Salsa:** Dice kiwi and combine with chopped tomatoes, onions, cilantro, jalapeno, lime juice, and a pinch of salt for a flavorful and refreshing salsa that pairs well with grilled fish or chicken.

4. **Kiwi Parfait:** Layer chopped kiwi with Greek yogurt, granola, and a drizzle of honey or maple syrup for a nutritious and satisfying parfait that's perfect for breakfast or dessert.

5. **Kiwi Sorbet:** Blend frozen kiwi with a splash of orange juice and a touch of honey or agave syrup until smooth, then freeze until firm for a refreshing and healthy dessert option.

Lentils Diet

Definition: The lentils diet involves incorporating lentils as a versatile and nutritious legume into meals to boost protein, fiber, vitamins, and minerals intake. Lentils are an excellent source of plant-based protein, making them a valuable addition to vegetarian and vegan diets.

Ingredients:

- **Lentils:** The star ingredient, rich in protein, fiber, vitamins (such as folate and vitamin B6), and minerals (such as iron and magnesium), serves as the foundation of this diet.

- **Vegetables:** Pair lentils with a variety of vegetables such as carrots, onions, tomatoes, spinach, or bell peppers for added flavor, texture, and nutrients.

- **Whole Grains:** Serve lentils alongside whole grains like brown rice, quinoa, or whole wheat couscous for added fiber and sustained energy.

- **Herbs and Spices:** Flavor lentil dishes with herbs, spices, and seasonings like garlic, cumin, coriander, or smoked paprika to enhance taste and aroma.

- **Healthy Fats:** Incorporate sources of healthy fats such as olive oil, avocado, nuts, or seeds to enhance satiety and nutrient absorption.

Instructions:

1. **Lentil Soup:** Simmer lentils with vegetables, broth, and seasonings to create a hearty and nutritious soup that's perfect for cold weather or when you're feeling under the weather.

2. **Lentil Salad:** Toss cooked lentils with mixed greens, chopped vegetables, herbs, nuts, seeds, and a vinaigrette for a

refreshing and satisfying salad that's packed with plant-based protein and fiber.

3. **Lentil Curry:** Cook lentils with coconut milk, tomatoes, onions, garlic, ginger, and curry spices for a flavorful and comforting curry dish that pairs well with rice or naan.

4. **Lentil Stew:** Combine lentils with root vegetables, tomatoes, broth, and herbs in a slow cooker or Instant Pot for a hearty and nourishing stew that's easy to prepare and perfect for meal prep.

5. **Lentil Tacos:** Fill taco shells or tortillas with seasoned lentils, lettuce, tomatoes, avocado, salsa, and a squeeze of lime for a tasty and nutritious meatless taco option that's suitable for vegetarians and vegans.

Mango Diet

Definition: The mango diet emphasizes the incorporation of mangoes as a primary source of vitamins, minerals, and antioxidants into meals or snacks. Mangoes are renowned for their high vitamin C content, as well as their fiber, vitamin A, and potassium, making them a delicious and nutritious addition to any diet.

Ingredients:

- **Mango:** The star ingredient, rich in vitamin C, vitamin A, fiber, and antioxidants, serves as the foundation of this diet.

- **Other Fruits:** Pair mango with other fruits such as berries, pineapple, or kiwi for added flavor, sweetness, and variety.

- **Greek Yogurt:** Combine mango with Greek yogurt for a creamy and nutritious breakfast or snack option that's rich in protein and probiotics.

- **Nuts and Seeds:** Sprinkle chopped mango over nuts or seeds like almonds, walnuts, or chia seeds for added texture, healthy fats, and nutritional variety.

- **Whole Grains:** Serve mango alongside whole grains like quinoa, brown rice, or whole grain toast for added fiber and sustained energy.

Instructions:

1. **Mango Smoothie:** Blend mango chunks into smoothies along with other fruits, leafy greens, Greek yogurt, nut milk, and a scoop of protein powder for a tropical and refreshing beverage that's packed with vitamins, minerals, and protein.

2. **Mango Salsa:** Dice mango and combine with chopped tomatoes, onions, cilantro, jalapeno, lime juice, and a pinch of salt for a flavorful and vibrant salsa that pairs well with grilled fish or chicken.

3. **Mango Salad:** Combine sliced mango with mixed greens, avocado, red onion, toasted nuts, and a citrus vinaigrette for

a refreshing and nutrient-rich salad that's perfect for summer.

4. **Mango Chia Pudding:** Mix pureed mango with chia seeds and almond milk, then let it sit in the fridge until thickened for a creamy and satisfying pudding that's rich in fiber, protein, and omega-3 fatty acids.

5. **Mango Sorbet:** Blend frozen mango chunks with a splash of coconut water or orange juice until smooth, then freeze until firm for a refreshing and healthy dessert option that's perfect for hot days.

Mushrooms Diet

Definition: The mushrooms diet involves incorporating mushrooms as a versatile and nutritious ingredient into meals to boost flavor, texture, and nutrient intake. Mushrooms are low in calories, fat-free, and rich in vitamins (such as vitamin D and B vitamins), minerals (such as selenium and potassium), and antioxidants.

Ingredients:

- **Mushrooms:** The star ingredient, rich in vitamins, minerals, and antioxidants, serves as the foundation of this diet.

- **Vegetables:** Pair mushrooms with a variety of vegetables such as onions, garlic, bell peppers, spinach, or tomatoes for added flavor, texture, and nutrients.

- **Whole Grains:** Serve mushrooms alongside whole grains like quinoa, brown rice, or whole wheat pasta for added fiber and sustained energy.

- **Proteins:** Pair mushrooms with proteins like chicken, tofu, beef, or seafood to create balanced and satisfying meals.

- **Herbs and Spices:** Flavor mushroom dishes with herbs, spices, and seasonings like thyme, rosemary, garlic powder, or smoked paprika to enhance taste and aroma.

Instructions:

1. **Mushroom Stir-Fry:**Saute sliced mushrooms with garlic, ginger, soy sauce, and your choice of protein for a quick and flavorful Asian-inspired dish that's perfect for busy weeknights.

2. **Stuffed Mushrooms:** Fill mushroom caps with a mixture of breadcrumbs, cheese, herbs, and spices, then bake until golden and crispy for a delicious and satisfying appetizer or snack.

3. **Mushroom Risotto:** Cook mushrooms with arborio rice, onions, garlic, white wine, and broth until creamy and tender for a comforting and luxurious risotto that's perfect for date night or special occasions.

4. **Mushroom Soup:** Simmer mushrooms with onions, celery, carrots, broth, and herbs until tender, then puree until

smooth for a rich and velvety soup that's perfect for cold weather.

5. **Grilled Mushroom Skewers:** Thread mushrooms onto skewers with bell peppers, onions, and cherry tomatoes, then grill until charred and tender for a flavorful and colorful side dish or vegetarian entree option.

Oatmeal Diet

Definition: The oatmeal diet involves incorporating oatmeal as a primary source of whole grains into meals to boost fiber intake and promote satiety. Oatmeal is rich in soluble fiber, vitamins, minerals, and antioxidants, making it a nutritious and filling option for breakfast or any time of the day.

Ingredients:

- **Oatmeal:** The star ingredient, rich in soluble fiber, vitamins (such as B vitamins), minerals (such as iron and magnesium), and antioxidants, serves as the foundation of this diet.

- **Liquid:** Cook oatmeal with liquids such as water, milk (dairy or plant-based), or fruit juice for added flavor, creaminess, and nutrition.

- **Fruits:** Pair oatmeal with fruits like berries, bananas, apples, or oranges for added flavor, natural sweetness, and additional vitamins and minerals.

- **Nuts and Seeds:** Sprinkle chopped nuts or seeds like almonds, walnuts, or chia seeds over oatmeal for added texture, healthy fats, and nutritional variety.

- **Sweeteners (Optional):** Add natural sweeteners like honey, maple syrup, or agave nectar if desired, but keep in mind the added sugar content.

Instructions:

1. **Basic Oatmeal:** Cook oatmeal according to package instructions, then serve with your choice of toppings such as fruits, nuts, seeds, and a drizzle of honey or maple syrup for a simple and satisfying breakfast option.

2. **Overnight Oats:** Mix oats with milk (or yogurt) and your choice of toppings in a jar or container, then refrigerate overnight for a convenient and portable breakfast option that's ready to eat in the morning.

3. **Oatmeal Pancakes:** Make pancakes using oatmeal as a base along with eggs, milk, and baking powder for a nutritious and hearty breakfast option that's perfect for weekends or special occasions.

4. **Baked Oatmeal:** Combine oats with milk, eggs, fruits, nuts, and spices, then bake until set for a delicious and comforting breakfast casserole that can be enjoyed warm or cold.

5. **Oatmeal Smoothie:** Blend cooked oatmeal with fruits, Greek yogurt, nut milk, and a scoop of protein powder for a creamy and filling smoothie that's perfect for post-workout recovery or as a meal replacement option.

THE END